AF904927

PRIMARY CARE IN PRACTICE - INTEGRATION IS NEEDED

Edited by **Oreste Capelli**

Primary Care in Practice - Integration is Needed
http://dx.doi.org/10.5772/59524
Edited by Oreste Capelli

Contributors

Jose María Arribas Blanco, Claire Collins, Oreste Capelli, Imma Cacciapuoti, Andrea Fabbo, Luc Pieter De Vreese, Silvia Riccomi, Lucia Borsari, Marco Vinceti, Monica Lorenzini, Valentina Solfrini, Federica Abate, Caterina Ricci, Barbara Casalgrandi, Letizia Reggianini, Gianbattista Spagnoli, Benedetta Quattrini, Eleonora Savi

Published by InTech

Janeza Trdine 9, 51000 Rijeka, Croatia

© The Editor(s) and the Author(s) 2016

The moral rights of the editor(s) and the author(s) have been asserted.
All rights to the book as a whole are reserved by InTech. The book as a whole (compilation) cannot be reproduced, distributed or used for commercial or non-commercial purposes without InTech's written permission. Enquiries concerning the use of the book should be directed to InTech's rights and permissions department (permissions@intechopen.com).
Violations are liable to prosecution under the governing Copyright Law.

Individual chapters of this publication are distributed under the terms of the Creative Commons Attribution 3.0 Unported License which permits commercial use, distribution and reproduction of the individual chapters, provided the original author(s) and source publication are appropriately acknowledged. More details and guidelines concerning content reuse and adaptation can be found at http://www.intechopen.com/copyright-policy.html.

Notice

Statements and opinions expressed in the chapters are these of the individual contributors and not necessarily those of the editors or publisher. No responsibility is accepted for the accuracy of information contained in the published chapters. The publisher assumes no responsibility for any damage or injury to persons or property arising out of the use of any materials, instructions, methods or ideas contained in the book.

Publishing Process Manager Iva Lipovic

Technical Editor InTech DTP team

Cover InTech Design team

First published May, 2016

Printed in Croatia

Additional hard copies can be obtained from orders@intechopen.com

Primary Care in Practice - Integration is Needed, Edited by Oreste Capelli

p. cm.

Print ISBN 978-953-51-2399-6
Online ISBN 978-953-51-2400-9

We are IntechOpen, the first native scientific publisher of Open Access books

3,350+
Open access books available

108,000+
International authors and editors

114M+
Downloads

151
Countries delivered to

Our authors are among the
Top 1%
most cited scientists

12.2%
Contributors from top 500 universities

WEB OF SCIENCE™

Selection of our books indexed in the Book Citation Index in Web of Science™ Core Collection (BKCI)

Interested in publishing with us?
Contact book.department@intechopen.com

Numbers displayed above are based on latest data collected.
For more information visit www.intechopen.com

For EU product safety concerns:
IN TECH d.o.o., Prolaz Marije Krucifikse Kozulić 3, 51000 Rijeka, Croatia,
info@intechopen.com or visit our website at intechopen.com.

Meet the editor

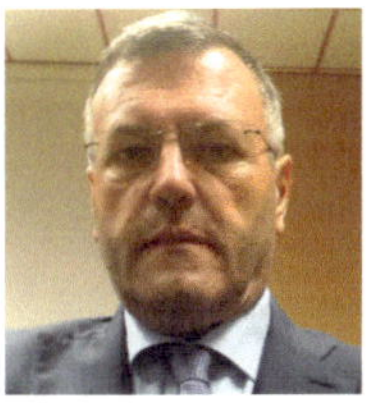

Dr. Oreste Capelli was born in 1956 in Bologna (Italy). After graduating in Medicine and Surgery at Modena University (1981), he became a specialist in Pneumology (1985) and Internal Medicine (1992). From 1985 to 1990, he worked at Modena University Hospital, teaching clinical methodology in the graduate school of pulmonary medicine. From 1991 to 2003, Dr. Capelli worked as a General Practitioner, collaborating with the Local Health Authority (LHA) to implement guidelines and clinical audit in the Community. In 2004, Dr. Capelli completed a Master in EBM and Research Methodology and then he worked for the Centre for the Evaluation of Effectiveness of Health Care (CeVEAS) at Modena LHA, as an "Audit and feedback" expert. After 2 years of experience (2012–2013), as a head of the Unit for Integrated Management of Chronic Diseases at the Regional Health Authority of Emilia-Romagna (Bologna, Italy), Dr. Capelli directs the Services' Epidemiology and Clinical Governance Unit of the Modena LHA.

Contents

Preface

The development of the Chronic Care Model (CCM) for the care of patients with chronic diseases has focused on the integration of taking charge of the patients and their family within primary care. The major critical issues in the implementation of the CCM principles are the non-application of the best practices, defined by EBM guidelines, the lack of care coordination and active follow-up of clinical outcomes, and by inadequately trained patients, who are unable to manage their illnesses.

The integrated care involves various different concepts and programs designed to promote coordination within and between healthcare organizations, with the goal of improving patient care, health outcomes, and boost the overall efficiency of healthcare systems.

This book focuses on these points: the value of an integrated approach to some chronic conditions, the value of the care coordination across the continuum of the illness, the importance of an evidence-based management, and the enormous value of the patients' involvement in the struggle against their conditions, without forgetting the essential role of the caregivers and the community when the diseases become profoundly disabling.

"Primary care, buttressed by appropriate specialty care, unifies a health system and focuses it on people's problems, not on specific diseases, whether they fit the current conceptualization of chronic illness or not." [1]

How can we fail to agree with the words of Barbara Starfield and her decades-long valorization of the primary care work? Her work showed that a robust primary care system guarantees the best care outcomes for prevention and care of chronic conditions and is able both to counteract the adverse effects of the low socioeconomic status to allow substantial welfare savings. [2]

I wish to dedicate this book to Barbara Starfield and to her clear thinking and tireless work for improving the health of millions of people around the world.

Barbara has left, but her thinking lives strong with us. Thank you!

Oreste Capelli, MD
Head, Services' Epidemiology and Clinical Governance Unit,
Modena Local Health Authority, Italy

1) Starfield B. Chronic illness, comorbidity, and primary care quality. In: Rosen B, Saltman R, Shani M. Health Systems: Are We in a Post Reform Era? Jerusalem: Israel National Institute for Health Policy and Health Services Research, 2006, pp. 81-84.

2) Starfield B. Benefits of Primary Care in Healthcare Reform, Herbert Vaughn Lecture, Boston 2010

Section 1

Integration in Primary Care: The Principles

Chapter 1

Integrated Care for Chronic Diseases – State of the Art

O. Capelli, B. Quattrini, F. Abate, B. Casalgrandi and I. Cacciapuoti

Additional information is available at the end of the chapter

http://dx.doi.org/10.5772/63362

Abstract

Chronic diseases represent a high cost for healthcare systems, for individuals, families, businesses and governments. The World Health Organization (WHO) estimates that an increase of 10% of chronic diseases is associated with a reduction of 0.5% of annual economic growth. Primary care has proven to ensure high levels of efficiency, effectiveness, equity, safety, timely and centrality of the patient achieving better health outcomes and lower costs. The Chronic Care Model (CCM) proposes a proactive approach in assisting the empowerment of patients and their community. The CCM contributes to improving the quality of care and health outcomes and the reduction of inequalities (e.g., ethnicity, social status) too.

The primary care team has the responsibility for coordination of care for patients living in the community. The teamwork integration is a crucial point. The integrated care involves various programs designed to promote coordination within and between health care organisations, with the aim to improve patient care and health outcomes and to boost the overall efficiency of health care systems. Scientific evidence shows that integrated care reduces the use of some resources (hospitalisations, emergency room visits, direct costs) in the management of chronic diseases, such as chronic heart failure, diabetes mellitus and chronic obstructive pulmonary disease. Vice versa, lack of integrated care risks making the care inappropriate, fragmented and/or redundant and at risk of errors. The integration of system activity in chronic disease management, entrusted to the primary care, must be transposed and implemented by all health professionals who follow the patient. Health professionals must organize care by adopting a patient-centred approach, supporting the paths of self-management and ensuring the exchange of information among both professionals and patients themselves and working in a public-health perspective. Continuity of care is one of the fundamental aspects of the integration programmes. Intermediate care and transitional care should assure the multi-professional coordination and cover the connection and the patient's transition between the various areas of assistance, between the hospital and the patient's home. Last but not least, integrated care needs the patient's involvement as an essential tool of the process.

INTECH
open science | open minds

© 2016 The Author(s). Licensee InTech. This chapter is distributed under the terms of the Creative Commons Attribution License (http://creativecommons.org/licenses/by/3.0), which permits unrestricted use, distribution, and reproduction in any medium, provided the original work is properly cited.

There is growing evidence that effective self-management is critical to optimising health outcomes for people with chronic diseases.

Keywords: Chronic diseases, integrated care, multimorbidity, continuity of care, primary care

1. Introduction

1.1. The epidemic of chronic diseases

In Western countries, the progressive increase in life expectancy in the general population and chronic diseases in the aged population has profoundly changed the scenario of health needs [1].

The World Health Organization (WHO) (2002) defines chronic diseases as "health problems that require an ongoing management over a period of years or decades, and include: diabetes, heart diseases, asthma, chronic respiratory diseases, cancer, HIV/AIDS, dementia, depression and physical disability " [2].

Chronic diseases represent a high cost for health care systems, for individuals, families, businesses and governments. The WHO estimates that an increase of 10% of chronic diseases is associated with a reduction of 0.5% of annual economic growth [3].

Globally, chronic conditions are the main causes of death in Western countries. For example, about two-thirds of the deaths that occurred in 2008 (36 million vs. 57 million) was attributable to chronic non-communicable diseases, including cardiovascular diseases (48% of chronic diseases), cancer (21%), chronic respiratory diseases (12%) and diabetes (3.5%) [3].

In the coming years, the prevalence of chronic diseases is estimated to increase rapidly, both due to the unrestrainable ageing process of the world population and the increased longevity of people with chronic pathologies [3–5]. A growing number of people has two or more diseases, interdependent (co-morbidities) or as co-occurrence of multiple diseases in the same individual (chronic multimorbidity) [1, 3, 6–10]. Multimorbidity is significantly associated with increased mortality and disability and a lower quality of life [9–10]. Its prevalence can be estimated at 20–30% of the general population and it rises from 55% to 98% when considering the elderly or disadvantaged social classes [7–10].

The spread of chronic diseases not only affects countries with a medium-high level of wealth, but also the countries with lower wealth levels [11], as evidenced by more than 80% of deaths from cardiovascular problems or diabetes, and almost 90% of those for chronic obstructive pulmonary disease (COPD), occurring in low- and middle-income countries.

According to the WHO greatest part of the human and social impact caused by chronic diseases could be prevented through transparent actions, efficient and sustainable [3], since a significant reduction of the impact of chronic diseases will depend more and more from preventive interventions that are going to systematically implement the entire population.

These interventions, easily available at low cost and high efficiency, should take into account, among different aspects, also the role of socio-economic inequalities, as the populations most affected by chronic diseases are also those with a greater condition of deprivation. Any policy should have a bio-psycho-social approach to prevent the burden of chronic diseases and should act on the inequalities of the social determinants of health (e.g., income, education, home, services, physical environment) [12].

Among the social determinants of health, health services have a relatively greater impact on the severity of illness (including death) rather than on their social impact. Since the inequalities on the severity of health problems (including disability, death and co-morbidity) are more relevant than inequality in the incidence of health problems, appropriate health services play an essential role in reducing inequalities in health" [13].

According to Margaret Chan, director of the WHO, in the health sector, **primary care** plays a privileged role in contrasting social inequalities in health: "The primary care is the best framework in which to act to ensure that all stakeholders, including the outside of the health sector, examine their impact on health".

The WHO has advocated for a long time an integrated approach in the prevention and the treatment of all chronic diseases. Key points of chronic management are represented by the existence of an efficient system of primary care and the development of the empowerment of patients and their caregivers.

From 2000 to 2010, the WHO has promoted several surveys to evaluate the capacity of prevention and control of chronic diseases in the Member States. The surveys have found that some progress has been made, but not in a uniform way, especially in high-income countries. Many countries are developing strategies, plans and guidelines for the fight against chronic diseases and risk factors.

In 2013, the WHO has proposed a multiannual action plan to be implemented over the period 2013-2020 for the prevention and control of chronic diseases, in particular cardiovascular diseases, cancers, chronic respiratory diseases and diabetes [3].

In the plan are highlighted six strategic objectives (Table 1), and, for each objective, a set of actions are outlined that all Member States and other international partners should achieve. The task of defining the priorities and establish strategic planning must be undertaken by a mixed team of primary care providers and community representatives.

The primary care, both in the report of the WHO (2008) "Primary Health Care: Now More Than Ever" [14] and in the Tallinn Charter, devoted to "Health Systems for Health and Wealth" (2008), [15] has proven to ensure high levels of quality in terms of efficiency, effectiveness, equity, safety, timely and centrality of the patient both at the macro level (policy, funding and regulation) and locally (organization and provision of services), achieving better health outcomes and lower costs.

To raise the priority accorded to the prevention and control of non-communicable diseases in global, regional and national agendas and internationally agreed development goals, through strengthened international cooperation and advocacy.
To strengthen national capacity, leadership, governance, multisectoral action and partnerships to accelerate countries' response for the prevention and control of non-communicable diseases.
To reduce modifiable risk factors for non-communicable diseases and underlying social determinants through the creation of health-promoting environments.
To strengthen and orient health systems to address the prevention and control of non-communicable diseases and the underlying social determinants through people-centred primary health care and universal health coverage.
To promote and support national capacity for high-quality research and development for the prevention and control of non-communicable diseases.
To monitor the trends and determinants of non-communicable diseases and evaluate progress in their prevention and control.

Table 1. WHO's strategic objectives for the prevention and control of chronic diseases (modified from [3])

As defined by time [16, 17] a "community-oriented" primary care is characterised by:

- A systematic assessment of the health needs of the population;
- Identifying community health needs;
- The implementation of systematic measures, with specific population groups involved (e.g., directed to the change in lifestyle or improvement of living conditions);
- Monitoring the impact of these interventions, to test the results achieved regarding population health.

The principles outlined above are the basis of different organisational models for the care of chronic diseases, all of which draw origin from the Chronic Care Model (CCM) developed in the late 90's in California [18, 19]. The model proposes a proactive approach to assisting oriented empowerment of the patient and the community (Figure1), as opposed to a reactive approach, based on the acute event expectation, typical of hospital care.

The CCM is based on six key issues:

1. **community resources:** mobilizing community resources to sustain patients' needs through volunteer groups, self-help groups, etc;
2. **health care organizations**: create a culture, organisation and mechanisms that promote safe and high quality;
3. **self-care:** in chronic diseases the patient becomes an active protagonist of care processes. We need to promote effective self-managed support strategies that include assessment, definition of objectives, plans of action, coping strategies, problem-solving, and follow-up;

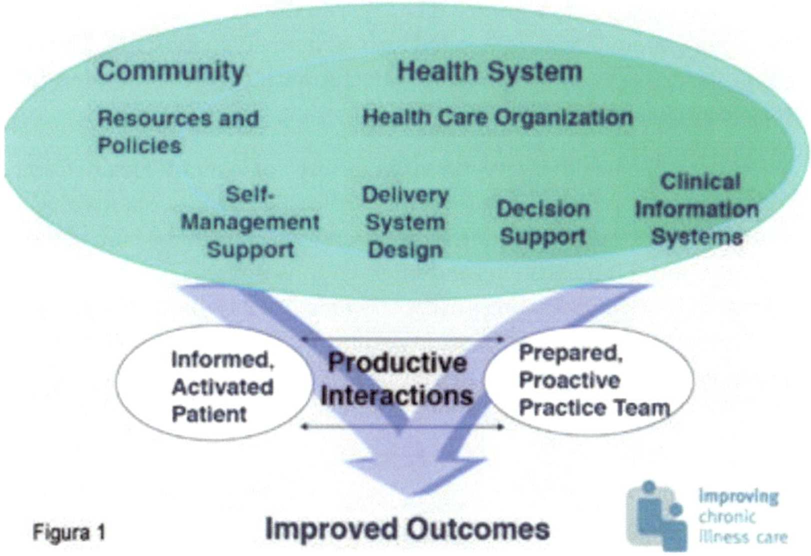

Figure 1. Chronic Care Model (reproduced with permission).

4. **The professional team:** the structure of the teamwork (specialists, general practitioners, nurses, educators) must be deeply modified, acting a clear division of activity and distinguishing assistance to acutely ill patients from the planned management of chronically ill patients;

5. **Decision support**: to promote care based on evidence and patient preferences; share guidelines and information with patients to encourage their participation.

6. **The development of computerized information systems**, which support three main functions:

   a. the pathology record keeping;

   b. alert system to support the primary care team to follow the guidelines;

   c. feedback for physicians, to monitor the performance of the team and the care system.

The CCM has been implemented in many countries, becoming an international reference model for the care of chronic conditions [5, 18, 20–34]. According to the available evidence, the CCM contributes improving the quality of care, health outcomes [30, 35] and the reduction of inequalities (e.g., ethnicity, social status) too [36].

2. Management of chronic diseases: integration is needed

The relevant changes in epidemiological profiles of the population, the socio-economic development of communities and family profiles [37], associated with remodelling in the care hospital network, impose equally significant changes in the way we deliver health and social care, through gripping models in an integrated load, as defined by the CCM. The paradigmatic example is the assistance provided to patients with chronic illnesses or multimorbidity, which require prolonged periods of assistance.

The effectiveness of public health interventions in the area of Primary Health Care is strongly linked to the development policies of the services and care activities that involve a high level of integration, both at the time of detection of needs and programming, both in the design and in services delivery, social interventions and interventions in the health area [38]. The ability to accurately identify the health resources necessary for subjects with multimorbidity and high care burden relies on the accuracy of measurements of risk adjustment that should address the problem in its entirety.

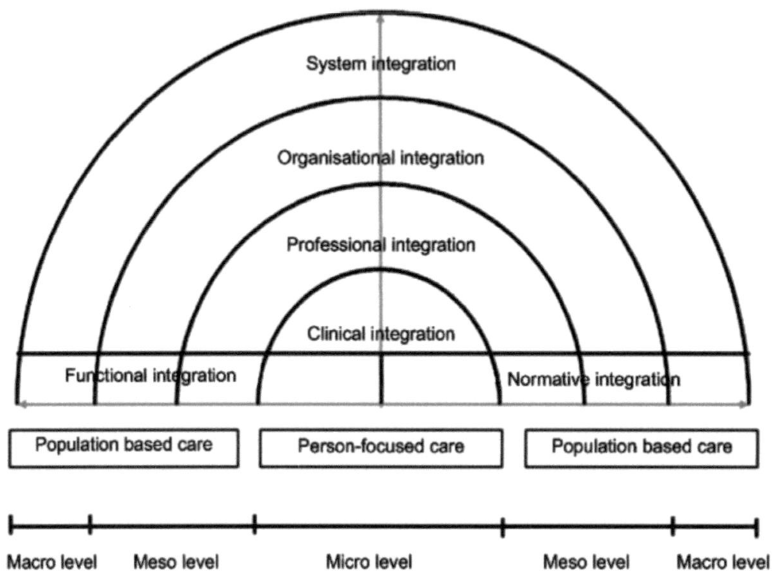

Figure 2. Conceptual framework for integrated care based on the integrative functions of primary care (reproduced with permission from Valentijn et al. [39]).

The major shortcomings in the management of chronic diseases include:

- Rushed practitioners not following established practice guidelines
- Lack of care coordination
- Lack of active follow-up to ensure the best outcomes
- Patients inadequately trained to manage their illnesses

It is essential to provide an organization that facilitates an integrated vision of health and social interventions. An integrated treatment system (Figure 2) based on the integrative function of primary care [39] includes multiple dimensions of integration, that have a complementary role on the micro level (clinical integration), meso (professional and organisational integration) and macro (system integration). The functional integration and the normative integration, however, guarantee the connection of all levels of a system.

Principle	Implementation example
1. Comprehensive services across the continuum of care	Integrated health systems are responsible from primary through to tertiary care and closely cooperate with social care organizations
2. Patient focus	Service planning and information management are driven by needs assessments and processes designed to improve patient satisfaction and outcomes
3. Geographic coverage and rostering	The system takes responsibility for a clearly defined population in a geographic area, but people can seek services from other providers if they wish
4. Standardized care delivery through inter-professional teams	Best practice guidelines, clinical care pathways and decision-making tools standardize and enhance quality of care; the use of electronic information systems facilitates effective communication
5. Performance monitoring	Monitoring systems measure care processes and outcomes at different levels and are linked to reward systems to promote the delivery of cost-effective high-quality care
6. Information systems	Computerized information systems allow effective tracking of utilization and outcome data across the continuum of care and serve consumers, payers and providers
7. Organizational culture and leadership	Committed leadership brings different cultures together, promotes the vision and mission of integration, and helps staff to take ownership of the process
8. Physician integration	Physicians are effectively integrated at all levels of the system and play leadership roles in the design, implementation and operation of the health system
9. Governance structure	Governance structures promote integration through representation of stakeholder groups involved in the delivery of healthcare along its continuum, including physicians and the community
10. Financial management	Financing mechanisms allow pooling of funds across services, for example, through global capitation, which pays for all insured health and some social services required by the enrolled population.

Table 2. Ten key principles for successful health systems integration (adapted from [40,44] with permission)

Lack of integration risks to make inappropriate the care processes, fragmented and/or redundant and at risk of errors. Despite a growing interest, to date a universally agreed definition of "integrated care" is still lacking [40]. In the literature, there are more than 180 definitions of terms and concepts relevant to one or more aspects of integration assistance. The integrated care involves a variety of different concepts and programs designed to promote coordination within and between health care organisations, with the aim to improve patient care, health outcomes and to boost the overall efficiency of health care systems. It is important to distinguish between integration and integrated assistance [41]:

- Integrated assistance is an organising principle of granting assistance;
- Integration describes necessary methods, processes and models to reach this kind of supply.

The experience of health care organisations that have achieved high levels of integration highlights the benefits that this kind of work can have for patients and, more generally, for the population [42–43].

A recent meta-review, referring to the ten key principles for evolved integrated systems (Table 2) showed that integrated care programs can improve the outcomes of patient-centred care, the quality of the processes and reduce the use of some health care resources (hospitalizations, emergency room visits, direct costs), in the management of chronic diseases such as chronic heart failure, diabetes mellitus and COPD [40].

3. The pivotal role of the Primary Health Care in an integrated health care system

Both the cited report "Primary Health Care: Now More Than Ever" [14] and the Tallinn Charter, devoted to "Health Systems for Health and Wealth" [15] defined the fundamental role of primary care in ensuring high levels of efficiency, effectiveness, equity, safety, timely and the patient's central role both at the macro level (policy, funding and regulation) and locally (organization and service delivery). More recently (2014) the European Commission, in light of the significant social and political changes mentioned above, decided to redefine the role of primary care, with special attention to the funding systems and referral. According to the panel's experts, Primary Care "... is the provision of universally accessible, integrated person-centred, comprehensive health and community services provided by a team of professionals accountable for addressing a large majority of personal health needs. These services are delivered in a sustained partnership with patients and informal caregivers, in the context of family and community, and play a central role in the overall coordination and continuity of people's care "[45].

The essential key concepts for the development of primary care, concern:

- **the community,** defined as a unit of a population that resides in a geographically defined territory, on which it has political and social responsibilities with everyday social interactions that cover all (or almost) the activities of daily living;
- **the role of patients**, with particular attention to the objectives defined by the patient regarding quantity and quality of life, and involvement in decisions about care (Shared Decision Making);
- **the role of informal caregivers** (e.g., family, friends, volunteers), to be interpreted as complementary, and not just as an extra that ensures the more formal (institutional) support;

http://dx.doi.org/10.5772/63362

- **an answer to most health problems**, which includes the full range of interventions, from the promotion of health care at the end of life, and that is related to the health sector as well as to the social sphere;
- **the integrated team work and the network of professionals** (including general practitioners, nurses, and social workers) who carry out their activities at a primary care centre or community hospital; this facilitates the work processes and inter-professional cooperation;
- **care coordination** with a central role given to the general practitioner;
- the enhancement of **the role of nurses** and other health professionals.

The primary care team, therefore, has the responsibility for coordination of care for patients living in the community. The Primary Health Care represents the privileged place to evaluate the patient's needs and oversee the paths of chronic patients, offering a proactive and personalised centre of services in integration and continuity with the offer of social policies. The identification, as early as possible, of individuals affected by or at increased risk of non-communicable chronic diseases and their subsequent take-over by the health care system is essential to reduce the risk of disability and mortality.

4. Population Health Management for chronic diseases

A population health approach focuses on improving the health status of the population. The action is directed at the health of an entire population, or subpopulation, rather than individuals. Focusing on the health of populations also necessitates the reduction in inequalities in health status between population groups.

As an approach, population health focuses on the interrelated conditions and factors that influence the health of populations over the life course, identifies systematic variations in their patterns of occurrence, and applies the resulting knowledge to develop and implement policies and actions to improve the health and well-being of those populations. [46, 47]

The Population Health Management approach represents, therefore, a cornerstone of the literature on chronic diseases and aims to maintain the population in good health by responding to the needs of individual patients both in terms of prevention and of treatment of chronic conditions through the identification of the target population based on health need, stratification by severity and assessment of take-over patterns (Figure 3).

To date, the Population Health Management [48] is a perspective, and not an exhaustive model, and that identifies a path of change articulated on six pillars:

1. Patient Population Identification
2. Health Assessment
3. Risk Stratification
4. Engagement

5. Patient-Centred Interventions
6. Impact Evaluation

Its purpose is the differentiation of the people affected or at risk of chronic diseases in sub-populations (sub-target) identified by complex care (disease staging) about the stage of development of the disease, the existence or absence of complications, specific requirements related to the coexistence of other diseases.

This differentiation results essential to define the most effective strategies and specific interventions tailored to the patients and to "customise" the care and treatment plan (Figure 4), respecting the patient's central role and his choices in the care pathway. It is also an essential prerequisite for efficiency by reducing the inappropriate interventions.

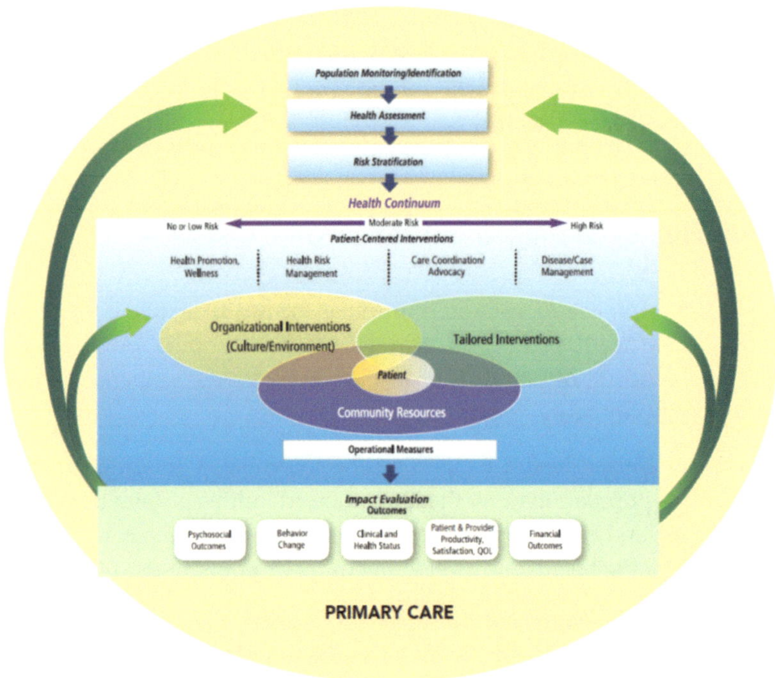

Figure 3. Population Health Conceptual framework (adapted with permission from [48]).

5. The competence of health workers involved in integrated care

The primary need to offer to patients clear and authoritative professional reference points along the care path can be resolved only by the conscious implementation of explicit management strategies shared by the various health professional and supported at the institutional level.

http://dx.doi.org/10.5772/63362

The integration of system activity in chronic disease management, entrusted to the primary care, however, must be transposed and implemented by all health professionals who follow the patient. The WHO has identified five fundamental competencies that health professionals need to apply for the treatment of chronic conditions (Table 3). [49]

Its purpose is the differentiation of the people affected or at risk of chronic diseases in sub-populations (sub-target) identified by complex care (disease staging) about the stage of development of the disease, the existence or absence of complications, specific requirements related to the coexistence of other diseases.

1. Patient-centred care
· Interviewing and communicating effectively
· Assisting changes in health-related behaviours
· Supporting self-management
· Using a proactive approach
2. Partnering
· Partnering with patients
· Partnering with other providers
· Partnering with communities
3. Quality improvement
· Measuring care delivery and outcomes
· Learning and adapting to change
· Translating evidence into practice
4. Information and communication technology
· Designing and using patient registries
· Using computer technologies
· Communicating with partners
5. Public health perspective
· Providing population-based care
· Systems thinking
· Working across the care continuum
· Working in primary health care-led systems

Table 3. Core competencies of the personnel assigned to take charge of patients with chronic diseases (adapted from [49])

This differentiation results essential to define the most effective strategies and specific interventions tailored to the patients and to "customise" the care and treatment plan (Figure

4), respecting the patient's central role and his choices in the care pathway. It is also an essential prerequisite for efficiency by reducing inappropriate interventions [48].

PHM Best Practice Level	1 Patient Population Identification	2 Health Assessment	3 Risk Stratification	4 Engagement	5 Patient-centered Interventions	6 Impact Evaluation
Level V	Clinician receives real-time, patient & population specific data at point of care	Clinician auto-notified of new or conflicting info requiring resolution	Valid tools auto- stratify patients & population across all clinicians; gaps flagged for action	"Medical home"; clinician monitors, optimizes care plan & care team across all settings	Clinician/Patient collaborative care plan; 1°, 2°, 3° prevention focus; coordinated team	Real-time feedback; outcomes meet & exceed patient , peer, population goals
Level IV	Patient information available from all clinicians - ID, risks, condition control	Patient health, values, preferences assessed; clinician receives info for consideration	Stratification lists available based on claims, HA, labs, screening info	Clinician engages with patient in "medical home," coordinates across connected settings	Clinician aware of & responds to patient needs/preferences focus on 1°, 2°, 3° prevention	Clinician receives patient outcome info; performance goals set in peer organization
Level III	Clinician registry – key diagnoses, tests, Hx, and condition control	Clinician evaluates health risks based on year-over-year comparing assessments	New health risks identified through health assessments and via registry lists	Clinician engages with patient focusing on both past and newly identified risks	Clinician focuses on 1°, 2°, 3° prevention; strategies for risks identified	Clinician unaware of patient outcome unless directly involved in care
Level II	Clinician has patient list with diagnoses	Clinician asks patients for baseline health assessment; assesses patient at the visit	Risk based on "frequent flier" status & clinician lists with diagnoses	Clinician engages with patient episodically at patient presentation	Intervention based on current patient need and known health risk(s)	Clinician unaware of patient outcome unless directly involved in care
Level I	Clinician identifies patient through direct interaction and hard-copy records	Clinician assesses patient at the visit	Clinician aware of high-risk patients based on "frequent flier" status	Clinician engages with patient episodically at patient presentation	Intervention based on current patient need and known health risk(s)	Clinician unaware of patient outcome unless directly involved in care

Figure 4. Population Health Conceptual framework (adapted with permission from [48]).

These skills, consistent with the provisions of the CCM organisational models, supplement those already acquired, such as the practice of care based on the evidence or attention to professional ethics.

Health professionals must organise care by adopting a patient-centred approach, supporting the paths of self-management and ensuring the exchange of information among both professionals and patients themselves and working in a public-health perspective.

6. Continuity of care in an integrated care system

The fragmentation of health care is one of the major risks to which the patient with multimorbidity is exposed [50]. If a unified vision of the health problem is lacking, there will frequently be a repetition of the traits of the common cure's path to more than one diseases, favouring a bureaucratic and economic burden.

Several studies have attempted to measure the continuity of cares in certain health professional areas (in particular, Mental Health and Family Medicine) or in certain categories of special need of complementing patients (basically, children and patients with chronic diseases).

The concept of continuity of care, as one of the fundamental aspects of the integration of care, has been studied thoroughly by Freeman [51] and Haggerty [52]. Although these studies did not achieve a unified definition and all-inclusive "continuity," a multidimensional classification of possible types of continuity of care in six logical categories has now been proposed:

1. Experienced continuity, defined as a set of relationships between the patient and one or more professionals coordinates from the health problem.

2. Continuity of information, based on the need of information exchange of the patient's clinical data.

3. Longitudinal continuity, the traditional definition of what constitutes the interpersonal relationship between the patient and one or more professionals who follow him/her over time.

4. Cross-boundary and continuity team, focused on the communication between professionals.

5. Flexible continuity, defined as the set of traders' efforts to make the flexible treatment process depending on the emergency

6. Interpersonal or relational continuity, defined as the set of interpersonal relations that exist not only between the patient and health professionals, but also among professionals who interact with the healing process.

This multi-dimensional definition [51] underpins some aspects of care continuity of relations among health professionals (medical and non-medical) who participate in the process of care for a particular patient and work together to exchange information about the health conditions of the patient [53]. This particular aspect of continuity, analysed by Freeman and Shepperd in a distinct way but complementary in the last three points of their multidimensional definition (i.e., cross boundary and continuity team, flexible continuity and interpersonal or relational continuity), is defined by the term "integration of care".

The concept of continuity has found development in other areas characterised by the need for integration of care and the information exchange between patient and one or more professionals: the family medicine, and in particular the paediatrician [54, 55], nursing care, especially in-home care, and care of people with chronic conditions [56, 57].

The potential benefits, traditionally ascribed by the literature to continuity of care, are essentially two [58, 59]:

a. **A greater satisfaction of the users of the system**, through the enhancement of interpersonal relationships structured in a way that are able to make more challenging the work for medical professionals and can increase the sense of care perceived by patients;

b. **A greater efficiency in the processes of care**, through a growing rationalisation of the treatment path (and, therefore, less risk of unnecessary duplication of benefits), lower transaction costs and lower information asymmetry.

7. Intermediate care for chronic diseases management

The concept of "intermediate care", born in England in 2000 in the National Beds Enquiry, has entered the lexicon of the European Health Policy. Over the years, in the literature, the delicate issue of integration between hospital and territory has been developed primarily with two perspectives:

1. The intermediate care, which covers all the intermediate areas of intervention between the hospital and the patient's home and that qualifies itself for multi-professional coordination [60–61];
2. The transitional care that concerns the manner of connection and the patient's transition between the various areas of assistance [62–65].

The intermediate cares, therefore, consist of an area of integrated services, both health and social, residential and domiciliary services, delivered in the context of primary care, where the care plan is actively agreed among health and social care professionals, patients and caregivers and where the patient's self-management is a primary goal. These services primarily aim to maximise the recovery of autonomy while keeping the patient as much as possible to his/her home and are provided by a multi-dimensional assessment of the patient, which supports an integrated and individualised plan of prevention and nursing. They are mainly intended for chronic patients and multi- morbidity. The care of the person with chronic conditions does not have by its very nature a result of healing, the concept of care, in fact, extends itself to interventions that allow a better living with the disease and the best residual function possible. Intermediate care can offer support to patients both in residential structures defined community hospital and at home, but it is still a limited service in time (no more than six weeks). The focus of these services is primarily rehabilitation, but with special attention also to the therapeutic management and self-education, ensuring continuity and coordination of the different services (health, social, etc.) and community resources.

8. The importance of self-management in the chronic diseases' integrated care

Self-management is the ability of the individual to manage the symptoms, the treatments, the life style changes and the psychosocial, cultural and spiritual consequences of the states of health [66]. Self-management is crucial in people with chronic diseases because the patient will be primarily responsible for their care throughout the course of the disease [67]. The orientation to the centrality of the assisted and self-determination presupposes a welfare approach and an organisation that considers the patient and his family, not only as active protagonists of the care processes, but also as subjects that need to be supported and oriented in the acquisition of skills necessary for the management and control of the disease(s).

The self-management of chronic disease has been recognized as a critical component of health cares for a long time; there is growing evidence that effective self-management is essential for optimising health outcomes for people with chronic diseases [68–82].

Patient education is focused on the patient's knowledge about his pathology in making the right decisions about his/her health and not just decisions about the disease, how the disease affects his/her role in working life, couple or social life, etc. [83].

http://dx.doi.org/10.5772/63362

In both European (e.g., Denmark, France, England, Sweden) and non-European (e.g., Australia, Canada, the United States) countries, structured programmes of **self-management of chronicity** have been implemented. Among others, there is the model of the Stanford University in California (Stanford chronic disease self-management program) also adopted in Australia (CDSMP), Canada and Europe.

The **Stanford Chronic Disease Self-Management Program** is a workshop, organised once a week, two and a half hours, for six weeks, in senior centres, libraries, churches and hospitals and attended jointly by people with different chronic conditions. Themes covered include:

- Techniques to deal with problems such as frustration, fatigue, pain and isolation
- Exercises to maintain and improve strength, flexibility and perseverance
- Appropriate use of medications
- Communicate effectively with family, friends, and caregivers
- Nutrition
- Evaluation of new treatments.

The workshops are run by two qualified leaders, with chronic diseases, one or both of whom are not health professionals [84].

9. Conclusions

The world of chronicity is an area in constant growth that involves a significant use of resources, requiring the guarantee of continuity of care for extended periods of time and a high multi-professional integration, both longitudinal (between hospital and territory) and transversal over the territory itself (between primary care and social services). The support of residential services (Hospice, community hospital, nursing home) is critical since they often are not sufficiently designed and developed even in the most advanced countries [85, 86].

The current "effective" treatments improve the prognosis, particularly in high-risk patients. The risk of survivors becomes increasingly higher with each new episode of exacerbation; the progression of the disease itself further increases this risk, with the need for new and more complex treatments, generating a "spiral" that only close with the patient's death [87].

Goals of care in patients with chronic illness, then not being able to be turned to healing, should be directed to the stabilisation as long as possible or to the improvement of their clinical conditions and their functional status, focusing on prevention of disabilities and maintaining the quality of life [88].

To achieve this, a high quality level of multi-professional and integrated care pathways is needed [89] in order to enable a long-term assistance of these chronic patients in their own homes with active participation of both the patients themselves and their caregivers, ensuring continuity of care and the best integration of social and health interventions [89–91].

Author details

O. Capelli[1*], B. Quattrini[1], F. Abate[1], B. Casalgrandi[1] and I. Cacciapuoti[2]

*Address all correspondence to: o.capelli@ausl.mo.it

1 Clinical Governance, Local Health Authority, Modena, Italy

2 Primary Health Care Department, Emilia-Romagna Region, Bologna, Italy

References

[1] Starfield B, Kinder K. (2011): Multimorbidity and its measurement. Health Policy. 2011 Nov;103(1):3–8. doi: 10.1016/j.healthpol.2011.09.004. Epub 2011 Oct 2.

[2] WHO, (2002): Innovative Care for Chronic Conditions: Building Blocks for Action.

[3] World Health Organization (2013): The European health report 2012: http://www.euro.who.int/__data/assets/pdf_file/0003/184161/The-European-Health-Report-2012,-FULL-REPORT-w-cover.pdf.

[4] Marengoni A, Winblad B, Karp A, Fratiglioni L. (2008): Prevalence of chronic diseases and multimorbidity among the elderly population in Sweden. American Journal of Public Health;98:1198–1200.

[5] de Bruin SR, Heijink R, Lemmens LC, Struijs JN, Baan CA. (2011): Impact of disease management programs on healthcare expenditures for patients with diabetes, depression, heart failure or chronic obstructive pulmonary disease: a systematic review of the literature. Health Policy. Jul;101(2):105–121. Epub 2011 May 18.

[6] Uijen AA, van de Lisdonk EH. (2008): Multimorbidity in primary care: prevalence and trend over the last 20 years. Eur J Gen Pract; 1: 28-32.

[7] Marengoni A, Angleman S, Melis R, Mangialasche F, Karp A, Garmen A, Meinow B, Fratiglioni L. (2011): Aging with multimorbidity: a systematic review of the literature. Ageing Research Reviews; 10:430–439.

[8] Jakovljević M, Ostojić L. (2013): Comorbidity and multimorbidity in medicine today: challenges and opportunities for bringing separated branches of medicine closer to each other. Medicina Academica Mostariensia; 1(1): 18–28.

[9] Barnett K, Mercer SW, Norbury M, Watt G, Wyke S, Guthrie B. (2012): Epidemiology of multimorbidity and implications for health care, research, and medical education: a cross-sectional study. Lancet; July 7; 380(9836):37-43. DOI:10.1016/S0140-6736(12):60240–60242.

[10] Boyd C, Fortin M. (2010): Future of multimorbidity research: how should understanding of multimorbidity inform health system design? Public Health Reviews; 32:451–474.

[11] WHO. (2005a): Preventing chronic diseases. A vital investment, ISBN 92 4 156300 1, http://www.who.int/chp/chronic_disease_report/contents/en/.

[12] WHO. (1997): Jakarta Declaration on Leading Health Promotion into the 21st Century The Fourth International Conference on Health Promotion: New Players for a New Era - Leading Health Promotion into the 21st Century, meeting in Jakarta from 21 to 25 July 1997: http://www.who.int/healthpromotion/conferences/previous/jakarta/declaration/en/.

[13] Department of Health, 2004, Improving Chronic Disease Management. http://www.dh.gov.uk/en/Publicationsandstatistics/Publications/PublicationsPolicyAndGuidance/DH_4075214.

[14] WHO, (2008), The World Health Report 2008, Primary Health Care: Now More Than Ever, ISBN 978 92 4 156373 4: http://www.searo.who.int/LinkFiles/Reports_whr08_en.pdf.

[15] Tallinn Charter: Health Systems for Health and Wealth, Copenhagen, (2008): WHO regional Office for Europe: http://www.salute.gov.it/imgs/C_17_pubblicazioni_1314_ulterioriallegati_ulterioreallegato_0_alleg.pdf.

[16] De Maeseneer J et al. (2007): Primary health care as a strategy for achieving equitable care, a literature review commissioned by Health Systems Knowledge Network, WHO.

[17] Maciocco G. (2012): Primary care, chronic diseases and the health rights. http://www.socialesalute.it/temi-in-discussione/cure-primarie-malattie-croniche-e-diritto-alla-salute.html.

[18] Wagner EH. (1998): Chronic disease management: what will it take to improve care for chronic illness? Eff Clin Pract; 1: 2–4.

[19] Bodenheimer T, Wagner EH, Grunbach K, (2002): Improving primary care for patients with chronic illness, JAMA; 288:1775–1779.

[20] Sperl-Hillen J, O'Connor PJ, Carlson RR et al. (2000): Improving diabetes care in a large health care system: an enhanced primary care approach. Jt Comm J Qual Improv; 26(11): 615–622.

[21] Fulton TR, Penney BC, Taft A. (2001): Exploring a chronic care model in a regional healthcare context. Healthc Manage Forum; 14(2): 6-24.

[22] Chin MH, Cook S, Drum ML et al. (2004): Improving diabetes care in midwest community health centers with the health disparities collaborative. Diabetes Care; 27(1): 2-8.

[23] Lozano P, Finkelstein JA, Carey VJ et al. (2004): A multisite randomized trial of the effects of physician education and organizational change in chronic-asthma care: health outcomes of the Pediatric Asthma Care Patient Outcomes Research Team II Study. Arch Pediatr Adolesc Med; 158.(9):875–883.

[24] Siminerio LM, Piatt G, Zgibor JC. (2005): Implementing the chronic care model for improvements in diabetes care and education in a rural primary care practice. Diabetes Educ; 31(2): 225–234.

[25] Stroebel RJ, Gloor B, Freytag S et al. (2005): Adapting the chronic care model to treat chronic illness at a free medical clinic. J Health Care Poor Underserved; 16(2): 286–296.

[26] Piatt GA, Orchard TJ, Emerson S et al. (2006): Translating the chronic care model into the community: results from a randomized controlled trial of a multifaceted diabetes care intervention. Diabetes Care; 29(4):811–817.

[27] Adams SG, Smith PK, Allan PF, Anzueto A, Pugh JA, Cornell JE. (2007): Systematic review of the chronic care model in chronic obstructive pulmonary disease prevention and management. Arch Intern Med. Mar 26;167(6):551–561.

[28] Peytremann-Bridevaux I, Staeger P, Bridevaux PO, Ghali WA, Burnand B.(2008): Effectiveness of chronic obstructive pulmonary disease-management programs: systematic review and meta-analysis. Am J Med;121(5):433-443.e4.

[29] Lewanczuk R. (2008): Hypertension as a chronic disease: what can be done at a regional level? Can J Cardiol. Jun;24(6):483–484.

[30] Coleman K, Austin B. T, Brach C and Wagner E.H. (2009): Evidence On The Chronic Care Model In The New Millennium, Health Affairs, 28, no.1 75-85:.http://content.healthaffairs.org/content/28/1/75.full.html.

[31] Nasmith L, Ballem P, Baxter R, Bergman H, Colin-Thomé D, Herbert C, Keating N, Lessard R, Lyons R, McMurchy D, Ratner P, Rosenbaum P, Tamblyn R, Wagner E, Zimmerman B. (2010): Transforming care for Canadians with chronic health conditions: Put people first, expect the best, manage for results - Appendices. Ottawa, ON, Canada: Canadian Academy of Health Sciences.

[32] Woltmann E, Grogan-Kaylor A, Perron B, Georges H, Kilbourne AM, Bauer MS. (2012): Comparative effectiveness of collaborative chronic care models for mental health conditions across primary, specialty, and behavioral health care settings: systematic review and meta-analysis. Am J Psychiatry. 1;169(8):790–804.

[33] Cramm JM, Nieboer AP. (2012): The chronic care model: congruency and predictors among patients with cardiovascular diseases and chronic obstructive pulmonary disease in the Netherlands. BMC Health Serv Res. 7;12:242.

http://dx.doi.org/10.5772/63362

[34] Chodosh J, Pearson ML, Connor KI, Vassar SD, Kaisey M, Lee ML, Vickrey BG. (2012): A dementia care management intervention: which components improve quality? Am J Manag Care; 18(2):85–94.

[35] Minkman M, Ahaus K, Huijsman R. (2007): Performance improvement based on integrated quality management models: what evidence do we have? A systematic literature review. Int J Qual Health Care. Apr;19(2):90-104. Epub. Review

[36] Nerenz DR. (2005): Health Care Organizations' Use Of Race/Ethnicity Data To Address Quality Disparities. Health Affairs; 2: 409–416.

[37] WHO-Europe (2013): Health 2020. A European policy framework and strategy for the 21st century.

[38] Starfield B. (2009): Primary care: an increasingly important contributor to effectiveness, equity, and efficiency of health services. Sespas report 2012. Gac Sanit, 26(Suppl 1):20–6.

[39] Valentijn P, Schepman SM, Opheij W, Bruijnzeels M. (2013): Understanding integrated care: a comprehensive conceptual framework based on the integrative functions of primary care. Int J Integr Care. 2013 Jan-Mar; 13: e 010.

[40] Martínez-González NA, Peter Berchtold P, Ullman K, Busato A, Egger M. (2014): Integrated care programmes for adults with chronic conditions: a meta-review. Int J Qual Health Care; 26(5):561-70.

[41] Shaw S, Rosen R, Rumbold B. (2011): What Is Integrated Care? A Research Report. London: Nuffield Trust.

[42] Curry N, Ham C. (2010): Clinical and service integration: the route to improved outcomes. London: The King's Fund. Available at: www.kingsfund.org.uk/publications/clinical-and-service-integration.

[43] Timmins N, Ham C. (2013): The quest for integrated health and social care: a case study in Canterbury, New Zealand. London: The King's Fund. Available at: www.kingsfund.org.uk/publications/quest- integrated-health-and-social-care.

[44] Suter E, Oelke ND, Adair CE et al. (2007): Health Systems Integration. Definitions, Processes & Impact: A Research Synthesis. Ottawa: Canadian Institutes of Health Research.

[45] Exph (Expert Panel on effective ways of investing in Health), 10 luglio 2014, Report on definition of a frame of reference in relation to primary care with a special emphasis on financing systems and referral systems. Available at: http://ec.europa.eu/health/expert_panel/opinions/docs/004_definitionprimarycare_en.pdf.

[46] Dunn JR, Hayes MV. (1999): Toward a lexicon of population health. Can J Public Health; Suppl 1(90):S7-S10.

[47] Kindig D, Stoddart G. (2003): What Is Population Health? Am J Public Health; 93(3): 380–383. PMCID: PMC1447747.

[48] Implementation and Evaluation: A Population Health Guide for Primary Care Models, (2012): Care Continuum Alliance: http://www.populationhealthalliance.org/publications/population-health-guide-for-primary-care-models.html.

[49] WHO, (2005): Preparing a health care workforce for the 21st century: the challenge of chronic conditions, ISBN 92 4 156280 3.

[50] Wolff JL, Giovannetti ER, Boyd CM, Reider L, Palmer S, Scharftstein D, Marsteller J, Wegener ST, Frey K, Leff B, Frick KD, Boult C. (2010): Effects of Guided Care on Family Caregivers. The Gerontologist; 50(4):459-470.

[51] Freeman G, Shepperd S, Robinson I, Ehrich K, Richards S. Continuity of care: report of a scooping exercise for the National Co-ordinating Centre for NHS Service Delivery and Organisation R&D (NHSCCSDO) London: NHSCCSDO; 2001. Available at: http://www.sdo.lshtm.ac.uk/continuityofcare.htm.

[52] Haggerty JL, Reid RJ, Freeman GK, Starfield BH, Adair CE, McKendry R. Continuity of care: a multidisciplinary review. BMJ 2003; 327:1219.

[53] Freeman G, Olesen P, Hjortdahl. (2003): P. Continuity of care: an essential element of modern general practice? Family Practice; 20 (6):623-627.

[54] Cassady CE, Starfield B, Hurtado MP, Berk RA, Nanda JP. Friedenberg LA. (2000): Measuring Consumer Experiences With Primary Care. Pediatrics ;105(4 Pt 2): 998-1003.

[55] Stewart AL, Grumbach K, Osmond DH, Vranizan K, Komaromy M, Bindman AB. (1997): Primary care and patient perceptions of access to care. J Fam Pract ; 44(2): 177-185.

[56] Freeman G. (1985): Priority given by doctors to continuity of care. J R Coll Gen Pract 35(278): 423–426.

[57] Rudebeck CE. (2002): Imagination and empathy in the consultation. Br J Gen Pract.; 52(479): 450–453. PMCID: PMC1314318.

[58] Becker MH, Drachman RH, Kirschit JP. (1974): A field experiment to evaluate various outcomes of continuity of physician care. Am J Public Health; 64(11): 1062–1070.

[59] Saultz JW. (2003): Defining and Measuring Interpersonal Continuity of Care. MD Ann Fam Med; 1(3):134–143

[60] Griffiths PD, Edwards MH, Forbes A, Harris RL, Ritchie G. (2007): Effectiveness of intermediate care in nursing-led in-patient units. Cochrane Database Syst Rev; 2:CD002214.

[61] Pearson MHH, Cooper C, Shepperd S, Pawson R, Anderson R. (2013): Intermediate Care: A Realist Review and Conceptual Framework. Final Report. Southampton:

NIHR Service Delivery and Organisation programme; Available at : http://www.netscc.ac.uk/hsdr/files/project/SDO_FR_10-1012-07_V01.pdf

[62] Hesselink G, Schoonhoven L, Barach P, Spijker A, Gademan P, Kalkman C, Liefers J, Vernooij-Dassen M, Wollersheim H. (2012): Improving patient handovers from hospital to primary care: a systematic review. Ann Intern Med;157(6):417–428. doi: 10.7326/0003-4819-157-6-201209180-00006.

[63] Philibert I, Barach P. (2012): The European HANDOVER Project: a multi-nation program to improve transitions at the primary care— inpatient interface. BMJ Qual Saf; 21:i1–6.

[64] Storm M, Siemsen IM, Laugaland KA, et al. (2014): Quality in transitional care of the elderly: key challenges and relevant improvement measures. Int J Integr Care;14:1–15.

[65] Centeno MM, Kahveci KL (2014): Transitional care models: preventing readmissions for high-risk patient populations. Crit Care Nurs Clin North Am;26(4):589-97. doi: 10.1016/j.ccell.2014.08.009. Epub 2014 Sep 16.

[66] Richard AA, Shea K. (2011): Delineation of self-care and associated concepts. Journal of Nursing Scholarship; 43:255–264.

[67] Lorig KR, Holman H. (2003): Self-Management Education: History, Definition, Outcomes, and Mechanisms, Ann Behav Med. 26(1):1-7.

[68] Wagner E.H., Austin B.T, Von Korff M.R. (1996): Organizing care for patients with chronic illness. Milbank Q 74(41):511–544.

[69] Von Korff M., Gruman J, Schaefer J, Curry SJ, Wagner EH. (1997): Collaborative management of chronic illness. Ann Intern Med; 127:1097–1102.

[70] Wagner EH, Glasgow RE, Davis C, Bonomi AE, Provost L, McCulloch D, Carver P, Sixta C. (2001): Quality improvement in chronic illness care: a collaborative approach. Jt Comm J Qual Improv. 27(2):63-80.

[71] Bodenheimer T, Lorig K, Holman H, Grumbach K. (2002): Patient self-management of chronic disease in primary care. JAMA 20; 288:2469–2475.

[72] Glasgow R.E, Funnell MM, Bonomi AE, Davis C, Beckham V, Wagner EH. (2002): Self-management aspects of the Improving Chronic Illness Care Breakthrough Series: Implementation with diabetes and heart failure teams. Ann Behav Med; 24:80–87.

[73] Glasgow R.E, Davis CL, Funnell MM, Beck A. (2003): Implementing practical interventions to support chronic illness self-management. Jt Comm J Qual Saf; 29:563–574.

[74] Gilbody S, Whitty P, Grimshaw J, Thomas R. (2003): Educational and organizational interventions to improve the management of depression in primary care: A systematic review. JAMA; 289:3145–3151.

[75] Brownson CA, Miller D, Crespo R, Neuner S, Thompson J, Wall JC, Emont S, Fazzone P, Fisher EB, Glasgow RE. (2007): A quality improvement tool to assess self-management support in primary care. Jt Comm J Qual Patient Saf; 33(7):408–416.

[76] Foster G, Taylor SJ, Eldridge SE, Ramsay J, Griffiths CJ. (2007): Self-management education programmes by lay leaders for people with chronic conditions. Cochrane Database Syst Rev; 17;(4):CD005108.

[77] Effing T, Monninkhof EM, van der Valk PD, van der Palen J, van Herwaarden CL, Partidge MR, Walters EH, Zielhuis GA. (2007): Self-management education for patients with chronic obstructive pulmonary disease. Cochrane Database Syst Rev; 17; (4):CD002990.

[78] Curtin RB, Walters BA, Schatell D, Pennell P, Wise M, Klicko K. (2008): Self-efficacy and self-management behaviours in patients with chronic kidney disease. Adv Chronic Kidney Dis; 15(2):191–205.

[79] Funnell MM. (2010): Peer-based behavioural strategies to improve chronic disease self-management and clinical outcomes: evidence, logistics, evaluation considerations and needs for future research. Fam Pract. 27 Suppl 1:i17-22.

[80] Battersby M, Von Korff M, Schaefer J, Davis C, Ludman E, Greene SM, Parkerton M, Wagner EH. (2010): Twelve evidence-based principles for implementing self-management support in primary care. Jt Comm J Qual Patient Saf; 36(12):561–570.

[81] Higgins R, Murphy B, Worcester M, Daffey A. (2012): Supporting chronic disease self-management: translating policies and principles into clinical practice. Aust J Prim Health; 18(1):80-87.

[82] Nolte S, Osborne RH. (2012): A systematic review of outcomes of chronic disease self-management interventions. Qual Life Res; 27. PMID: 23184454.

[83] Santurri LE. (2006): Patient Empowerment: Improving the Outcomes of Chronic Diseases Through Self Management Education. The MPHP 439 Online Text Book. Cleveland, Ohio: Case Western Reserve University.

[84] Chronic Disease Self-Management Program (Better Choices, Better Health® Workshop) http://patienteducation.stanford.edu/programs/cdsmp.html.

[85] Gonçalves-Bradley DC1, Lannin NA, Clemson LM, Cameron ID, Shepperd S. (2006): Discharge planning from hospital. Cochrane Database Syst Rev ; 1:CD000313. doi: 10.1002/14651858.CD000313.pub5.

[86] Aubin M, Giguère A, Martin M, Verreault R, Fitch MI, Kazanjian A, Carmichael PH. (20112): Interventions to improve continuity of care in the follow-up of patients with cancer. Cochrane Database of Systematic Reviews; Issue 7. Art. No.: CD007672. DOI: 10.1002/14651858.CD007672.pub2.

[87] O'Malley AS1, Rich EC, Maccarone A, DesRoches CM, Reid RJ. (2015) Disentangling the Linkage of Primary Care Features to Patient Outcomes: A Review of Current Lit-

erature, Data Sources, and Measurement Needs. J Gen Intern Med.; Aug 30 Suppl 3:S576-85. doi: 10.1007/s11606-015-3311-9.

[88] Smith SM, Soubhi H, Fortin M, Hudon C, O'Dowd T. (2012): Interventions for improving outcomes in patients with multimorbidity in primary care and community settings. Cochrane Database of Systematic Reviews; Issue 4. Art. No.: CD006560. DOI:10.1002/14651858.CD006560.pub2.

[89] Smith SM, Allwright S, O'Dowd T. (2007): Effectiveness of shared care across the interface between primary and specialty care in chronic disease management. Cochrane Database Syst Rev; (3):CD004910.

[90] Zwarenstein M1, Goldman J, Reeves S. (2009): Interprofessional collaboration: effects of practice-based interventions on professional practice and healthcare outcomes. Cochrane Database Syst Rev; (3):CD000072. doi: 10.1002/14651858.CD000072.pub2.

[91] Wallace E, Salisbury C, Guthrie B, Lewis C, Fahey T, Smith SM. (2015): Managing patients with multimorbidity in primary care. BMJ; 350:h176 doi: 10.1136/bmj.h176.

Chapter 2

Promoting Self-Management and Patient Empowerment in Primary Care

Claire Collins and Andree Rochfort

Additional information is available at the end of the chapter

http://dx.doi.org/10.5772/62763

Abstract

The complexity of health care is increasing, associated with several factors including aging populations and expanding comorbidities, growth in options for health interventions and patients' access to information from electronic and other media. Management of chronic conditions with high morbidity such as diabetes, cardiovascular disease, cancer, chronic pulmonary disease and depression constitutes a major burden of clinical care worldwide and an increasing problem for primary care because responsibility for chronic care shifts from hospitals to health professionals in primary care. Recently, there has been increasing attention focussed on another player/stakeholder in this quest to improve patient outcomes–the patient.

As of 9 September 2011, the new World Organization of National Colleges, Academies and Academic Associations of General Practitioners/Family Physicians (WONCA) EU definition of general practice includes as its 12th characteristic "Promotion of patient empowerment and self-care", following evidence of its relevance and importance.[1, 2]

During the course of a systematic review of the literature on the impact of health professional training regarding patient self-management on patient outcomes, we created a repository of information around the topics of patient self-management and empowerment. In this chapter, we synthesise this literature.

The systematic review was performed for articles published in advance of 1 September, 2013 using PubMed, ERIC, EMBASE, CINAHL, PsycINFO, Web searches, Hand searches and Bibliographies employing 13 search terms.

In conclusion, we note that there is a need to explore and to clarify the various aspects of patient empowerment and the many sources influencing successful patient self-management. These concepts involve a complex interaction of patient factors, health professional factors, health system factors and multiple other influences that need to be harnessed effectively by all stakeholders.

Keywords: Self management, patient empowerment, general practice, primary care, chronic conditions

INTECH
open science | open minds

© 2016 The Author(s). Licensee InTech. This chapter is distributed under the terms of the Creative Commons Attribution License (http://creativecommons.org/licenses/by/3.0), which permits unrestricted use, distribution, and reproduction in any medium, provided the original work is properly cited.

1. Introduction

The complexity of health care is increasing, associated with several factors including aging populations and expanding comorbidities,[3] growth in options for health interventions and patients' access to information from electronic and other media. Management of chronic conditions with high morbidity such as diabetes, cardiovascular disease, cancer, chronic pulmonary disease and depression constitutes a major burden of clinical care worldwide and an increasing problem for primary care as responsibility for chronic care shifts from hospitals to health professionals in primary care. Chronic diseases, often now referred to as non-communicable diseases, are of long duration and generally of slow progression.[4] Chronically ill individuals are more likely to have limitations in their daily living activity than others.[5] Chronic disease accounts for a significant proportion of the disease burden and an increasing workload for GPs, accounting for up to 60% of visits by patients 45 years and older.[6] The World Health Organisation (WHO) expects that chronic conditions will account for 73% of all deaths and 60% of morbidity and disability by 2020 and considers that one of the greatest challenges facing health care systems globally is the increasing burden of chronic diseases.[7] Multimorbidity, polypharmacy, complexity and increasing fragmentation of the management of chronic conditions are real challenges for GPs today. This complexity and fragmentation are reported by both patients [8, 9] and health care workers.[10, 11] Patients with multiple chronic diseases experience unfavourable health outcomes and give rise to challenges in patient care and medical costs.[12] It must be acknowledged that increasing demands and associated costs on health care system are not sustainable.

The availability of sufficient time for clinicians to manage a range of chronic conditions[13, 14] within the normal consultation time has been identified as a factor along with infrequent care coordination[15-17] and lack of active follow up.[10, 18-21] Furthermore, chronic illness requires a different approach from clinicians than acute illness.[22]

The WHO has suggested that the following skills are both useful and necessary to better manage chronic illness[23]:

a. Patient centred care — care needs to be organised to include patient involvement.

b. Quality improvement — measuring care and its outcomes, learning and adapting to change and translating evidence into practice.

c. Collaboration — partnering with patients, other health care workers/providers and communities.

d. Information and communication technology — designing and using patient registers, using computer technologies to support care and communicating with partners.

e. Public health perspective — health care workers need to broaden their perspective on health. This includes a better understanding of population-based care and the care continuum.

Battersby and colleagues[22] have expanded this list of core factors influencing primary health care workers (HCWs) and listed them in three domains: general patient-centred capabilities, behaviour change capabilities and organisational infrastructure.

While most GPs describe their approach as patient-centred, the latter does include elements that are sometimes missing in the doctor–patient relationship. There are five domains to patient-centred care.[24-26] These include the following:

- a biopsychosocial perspective
- patient-as-person
- sharing power and responsibility
- therapeutic alliance (establishing common ground)
- doctor as person.

Teasing these concepts out, Stewart[27] summarised the key elements of patient-centred care that are desired by patients. These include the following:

- an exploration of the patient's main reason for the visit, including their concerns and need for information
- an integrated understanding of the patient's world–that is, their whole person, including their emotional and other needs and life issues
- an attempt to find common ground on what the problem is and mutually agree on what should happen
- a greater role for prevention and health promotion
- strategies that enhance the continuing relationship between the patient and the doctor.

Others have suggested the use of 'person-centred care' to emphasise the importance of the doctor–patient relationship, which includes more reflection and an acknowledgement of the patient in his/her individual context as a person, and not simply as a patient.[28]

Wagner and colleagues[29] first described the chronic care model (CCM).[29] The chronic care model (Figure 1) is designed to make patient-centered, evidence-based care easier to achieve. The aim of the CCM is to transform the daily care for patients with chronic illnesses from acute and reactive to proactive, planned and population-based. It is designed to accomplish these goals through a combination of effective team care and planned interactions: self-management support including more effective use of community resources; integrated decision support and patient registers and use of other information technology (IT) resources. These elements are designed to work together to strengthen the clinician–patient relationship and improve health outcomes. Patient focussed care needs to include outcomes that are meaningful and helpful for the patient.[30] A wide range of interventions to improve patient outcomes in chronic illness have been implemented at health policy level, organisational level and health professional level. Interventions are targeted at secondary prevention to minimise complications as there is no absolute 'cure' for chronic conditions once established. Recently, there has been increasing attention focussed on another player in this quest to improve patient outcomes and that player or stakeholder is the patient. Patient participation in the management of their illness is now recognised as a factor that can improve patient outcomes and is a factor in implementing improvement in quality and safety of health care.[31]

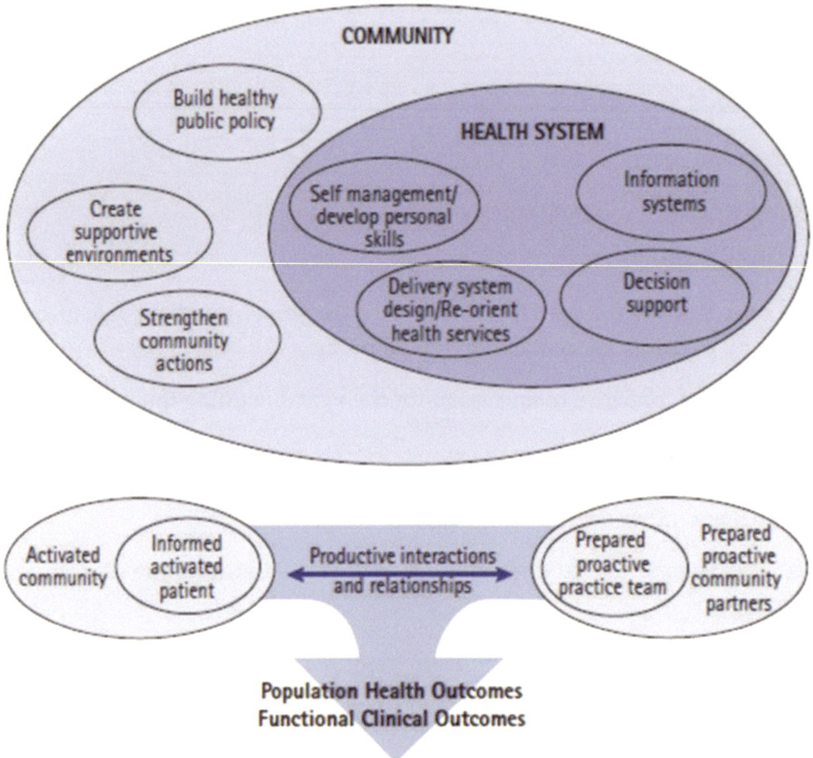

Created by: Victoria Barr, Sylvia Robinson, Brenda Narin-Link, Anita Dotts and Dariana Ravensdale (2002). Adapted from R. Glasgow, C. Orleans, E. Wagner, S. Curry and L. Solberg (2001). Does the Chronic Care Model also serve as a template for improving prevention? The Millbank Quarterly, 79(4), and World Health Organisation, Health and Welfare Canada and Canadian Public Health Association (1986). Ottawa Charter of Health Promotion. (This diagram may be found in Barr, Robinson, Marin-Link, Underhill, Dotts, Ravensdale & Salivaras, 2003.)

Figure 1. The chronic care model.

As of 9 September 2011, the new WONCA (*World Organization of National Colleges, Academies and Academic Associations of General Practitioners/Family Physicians)* European definition of general practice includes "Promotion of patient empowerment and self-care" as its 12th characteristic, following evidence of its relevance and importance. [1, 2, 32-34] The literature search by Mola et al.[32] provides evidence to support the specific setting of family medicine/general practice within the primary care setting as the optimum health care environment above other health care environments for promotion of patient empowerment and self-care. This is the basis of this newly accepted characteristic of patient empowerment being adopted as a core characteristic of the discipline of general practice rather than hospital-based care (Figure 2). Following adoption of this new characteristic, WONCA, through it anniversary grant, funded a collaborative project comprising of a systematic review and the creation of a template e-learning module focussing on patient self-management, of which patient empowerment is a key factor.

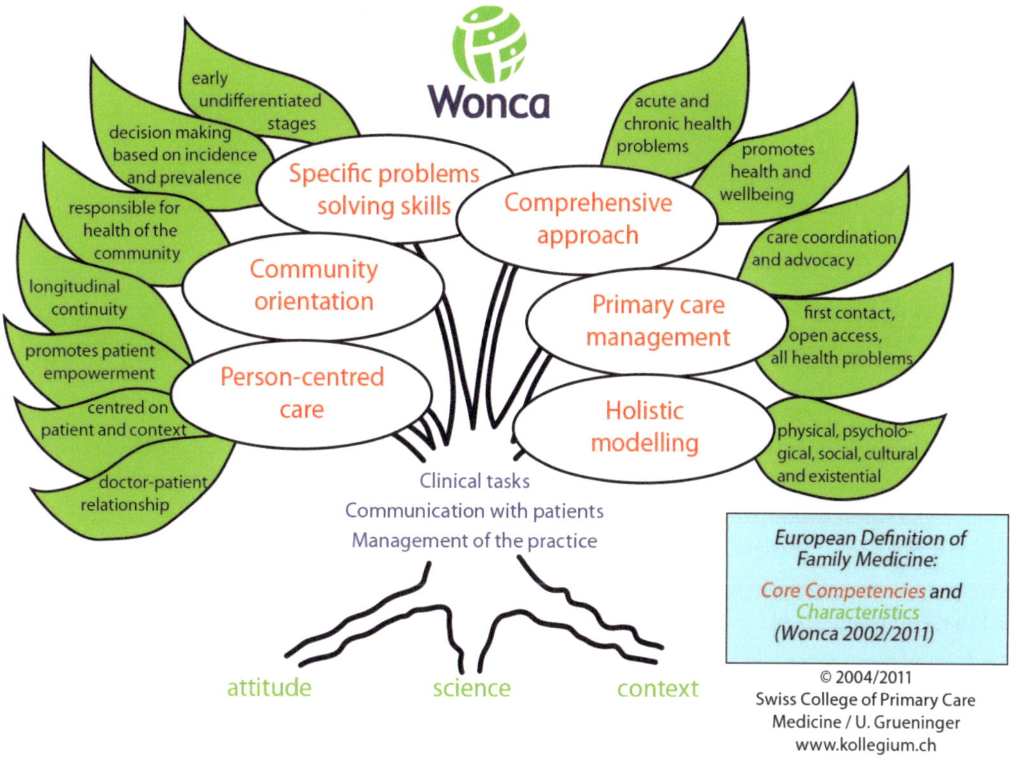

Figure 2. The WONCA tree.

While undertaking the systematic review, which focused on the impact of health professional training regarding patient self-management on patient outcomes (PROSPERO registration number: CRD42013004418), we created a repository of information around the topics of patient empowerment and self-management. In this chapter we synthesise this literature.

2. Methods

The systematic review was performed for articles published before 1 September 2013 using the following: PubMed, ERIC, EMBASE, CINAHL, PsycINFO, Web searches, Hand searches and Bibliographies employing the following search terms:

1. Primary healthcare
2. Physicians, primary
3. Physicians, Family
4. General Practitioners
5. #1 OR #2 OR #3 OR #4 NOT dental NOT pharma*
6. Education, continuing OR evidence-based medicine/education
7. Patient education as topic
8. Training
9. #6 OR #7 OR #8
10. "long term care"
11. Chronic disease
12. #10 OR #11
13. #5 AND #9 AND #12

All abstracts were reviewed using the RefWorks package to categorise the abstracts identified by the search. Articles not considered directly relevant to the systematic review where retained to populate a separate repository of information on subtopics. The key generic articles located from this search under the topics of patient self-management and patient empowerment and are synthesised in this chapter.

2.1. Self-management

Self-management, in the context of non-communicable disease, can be conceptualised as a set of tasks and processes that are used by a patient to maintain wellness in the presence of an ongoing illness.[35] Chronic condition self-management has been defined in numerous different ways; one example is: a process that includes a broad set of attitudes, behaviours and skills. It is directed toward managing the impact of the disease or condition on all aspects of living by the patient with a chronic condition. It includes, but is not limited to, self-care and it may also encompass prevention.[36]

A Cochrane Collaboration report[37] showed that improving patient self-management is one of the four categories of practice change that result in maximum impact on improving patient outcomes: the four categories being increasing clinicians' expertise and skill, educating and supporting patients, emphasis on team-based care delivery and making better use of IT-based patient registers.

Effective self-management skills can improve patient self-efficacy and reduce health care costs through fewer outpatient visits[38] and hospital admissions.[15, 39] Health professional training is associated with better uptake, implementation and effectiveness of self-management programs.[36, 40]

Self-management support is defined as the systematic provision of education and supportive interventions by health care staff to increase patients' skills and confidence in managing their health problems, including regular assessment of progress and problems, goal setting and problem-solving support.[41] Self-management support involves the application of collaborative goal setting and a range of self-efficacy strategies, for example, effective problem solving, monitoring his/her own condition, relapse prevention plans, patient education, group supports and shared decision making.[42]

Self-management support is the least implemented of the elements of the CCM[43] and has its own set of challenges, including developing and refining clinician skills in chronic care management, clinician self-efficacy and changing clinician behaviour. It is easy for clinicians to overlook the fact that many patients do not feel 'sick' with chronic conditions such as hypertension, diabetes or obesity.[44] Willcox and Gill[45] revealed uncertainty and a lack of understanding among health professionals regarding the concept of self-management support and its application. There is evidence available showing the efficacy of self-management support.[46-48]

Patient self-care affects health outcomes through numerous pathways,[49] such as follows:

- adherence to therapeutic regimens
- maintenance of health-related behaviours, e.g., lifestyle choices
- (self)-monitoring symptoms to inform treatment/self-care decisions
- monitoring and managing the emotional consequences of illness
- influencing the nature of communication between health care worker and patient to ensure that patients' needs are expressed and addressed
- using support networks to help achieve the above.

Self-management expands self-care with strategies to enhance the patient's own effectiveness and self-determination.[50] It requires greater collaboration with health care workers. An increasing number of patients are requesting a greater emphasis on shared care.[51-54]

Chronic care programmes that encourage self-management have been shown to be effective in a range of chronic diseases.[19, 20, 48, 55, 56-59] Improving specific patient and clinician behaviours (patient self-management and close monitoring of disease control parameters to achieve individualised goals) can improve disease control and quality of life among patients with multiple conditions and complex health care needs.[60]

Self-management methods promoted by primary care professionals should be based on best available evidence on effectiveness, safety and cost-effectiveness. Numerous system factors, patient factors and clinician factors influence effective patient self-management. System support for patient self-management (e.g., adequate time, training, IT, resources and support) is thought to contribute to an effective self-management process.[30]

Initiatives that both support patients and equip health professionals are required because each has a different function and both are required if self-management support is to be effective and sustainable.[16, 61] In terms of patient factors, coordination of methods to address barriers to patients' behaviour change is also key to successful patient self-management.[22] Two clinician factors, which might adequately be addressed at the level of continuing medical education and post-graduate training, are guideline non-adherence and sharing decision making with the patient; both require patient participation and engagement.[60, 62] Skill development in shared decision making can be incorporated into post-graduate professional development programmes and has been recommended.[63]

The educational focus around self-management needs to extend to all health care professionals in both primary and secondary services to ensure patients receive consistent and effective messages appropriate for their condition across the sector.[15] In the United Kingdom, the WISE (Whole System Informing Self-management Engagement) model advocates at patient, health care professional and structure of health care levels to support self-management practices.[64]

2.2. Patient empowerment

The idea of empowerment was first introduced in the 1960s by the Brazilian pedagogue Paulo Freire[1] and, with health care, has been acknowledged as an alternative to compliance to guide the provider–patient relationship.[65] Most patient empowerment definitions focus on individuals' capacity to make decisions about their health (behaviour) and to have, or take control over, aspects of their lives that relate to health[66] with most incorporating some form of personal control and self-efficacy/self-mastery.[35, 65, 67-71] Empowerment occurs when the health care professional's goal is to increase patients' capacity to make autonomous, informed decisions, and patients are making these decisions and choosing personally meaningful, realistic goals.[72]

Patient empowerment suggests more collaborative models of clinician–patient interaction. McAllister et al.[66] compared the paternalist and empowerment paradigms and suggested that the concept of empowerment could be another conceptualisation of the capability paradigm suggested by Sen.[73] A key attribute of patient empowerment is that the patient is not a passive recipient of health care and is self-determining with some control of his/her own health and health care.[35, 65, 69-71] However, Anderson et al.[74] argued that patients who choose to hand over responsibility should still be considered empowered being responsible for their choice, if not for their treatment.

Studies of patient empowerment in general practice and primary care to improve management of chronic diseases have shown good results, increasing patient and health professionals' satisfaction, adherence to guidelines and treatment and improving clinical outcomes.[1] With regard to success, research has indicated that multifaceted interventions are more effective than simpler ones[75] and that enduring change requires a multilevel approach,[76] with interventions at different levels interlinked and mutually reinforcing. This requires a whole systems perspective that involves interventions at the patient, practitioner and service organisation levels in the delivery of self-management support.

Although many factors (such as culture, age and socio-economic resources) influence empowerment, it is argued that empowerment can be considered to be either a process or an outcome and that patients can be empowered by their health care providers.[77, 78] As the concept of

http://dx.doi.org/10.5772/62763

patient empowerment continues to be the subject of further exploration, we can expect more refinement of its definition and relevance to patient health outcomes in primary care in the future.

General practice/family medicine (GP/FM) has been shown to be a suitable setting for promoting patient empowerment, because many of the characteristics of GP/FM are already oriented towards encouraging patient empowerment longitudinally over time. By its nature, primary care provides continuous, comprehensive and coordinated care across the care continuum.[79] The GP is in a key position to utilise and to promote patient and carer use of relevant information technology in patient empowerment. Tools such as personal health records (PHRs) integrated with electronic health records, interactive tools for health coaching, decision aids and decision support for both health professionals and patients are developing rapidly.[80] However, in order to effectively translate empowerment into clinical practice, will require health-care providers to adopt a truly patient-centred approach.[65]

3. Concluding remarks

Physicians can learn to be experts in management of medical conditions, but only patients can be experts in the conduct of their own lives.[81]

The patient has a role to play in determining his/her own health outcomes.[82] For optimum patient outcomes, there is a need to explore and to clarify for the clinician the various aspects of patient empowerment and the many sources of influence on successful patient self-management. These concepts involve a complex interaction of patient factors, health professional factors, health system factors and multiple other influences that need to be harnessed effectively by all stakeholders.

Author details

Claire Collins* and Andree Rochfort

*Address all correspondence to: claire.collins@icgp.ie

Irish College of General Practitioners, Dublin, Ireland

References

[1] Mola, E. Patient empowerment, an additional characteristic of the European definitions of general practice/family medicine. Eur J Gen Pract. 2013 Jun;19(2):128-31. doi: 10.3109/13814788.2012.756866. Epub 2013 Jan 22.

[2] WONCA Europe, 2011 Edition. Available online: http://www.woncaeurope.org/sites/default/files/documents/Definition%203rd%20ed%202011%20with%20revised%20wonca%20tree.pdf. [Accessed 2nd March 2016].

[3] Wallace, E., Salisbury, C., Guthrie, B., Lewis, C., Fahey, T., Smith, S.M. Managing patients with multimorbidity in primary care. *BMJ*. 2015 Jan 20; 350:h176. doi: 10.1136/bmj.h176.

[4] World Health Organization. *Health Topics: Noncommunicable diseases*. Available online: http://www.who.int/topics/noncommunicable_diseases/en/. [Accessed 2nd March 2016].

[5] Bhattacharya, J., Choudhry, K., Lakdawalla, D. Chronic disease and severe disability among working-age populations. *Med Care* 2008 Jan;46(1):92-100.

[6] Britt H, Miller GC, Charles J, Henderson J, Bayram C, Harrison C, Valenti L, Fahridin S, Pan Y, O'Halloran J 2008. General practice activity in Australia 1998–99 to 2007–08: 10 year data tables. General practice series no. 23. Cat. no. GEP 23. Canberra: Australian Institute of Health and Welfare. http://www.aihw.gov.au/WorkArea/DownloadAsset.aspx?id=6442456228.

[7] World Health Organization. Innovative care for chronic diseases. Building blocks for action. Global Report. Geneva: WHO, 2002.

[8] Walter, U., Flick, U., et al. Putting prevention into practice: qualitative study of factors that inhibit and promote preventive care by general practitioners, with a focus on elderly patients. *BMC Fam Pract*. 2010 Sep 20; 11: 68. doi: 10.1186/1471-2296-11-68.

[9] Yen, L., Gillespie, J., et al. (2011). Health professionals, patients and chronic illness policy: a qualitative study. *Health Expect* 2011 Mar; 14(1):10-20. doi: 10.1111/j.1369-7625.2010.00604.x.

[10] Ouwens, M., Wollersheim, H., et al. Integrated care programmes for chronically ill patients: a review of systematic reviews. *Int J Qual Health Care* 2005 Apr; 17(2):141-6. Epub 2005 Jan 21.

[11] Glasgow, N.J., Jeon, Y.H., et al. Chronic disease self-management support: the way forward for Australia. *Med J Aust* 2008 Nov 17; 189 (10 Suppl):S14-16.

[12] Parekh, A.K., Barton, M.B. The challenge of multiple comorbidity for the US health care system. *JAMA* 2010 Apr 7;303(13):1303-4. doi: 10.1001/jama.2010.381.

[13] Ostbye, T., Yarnall, K., et al. Is there time for management of patients with chronic diseases in primary care? *Ann Fam Med 2005;*2005 May-Jun; 3(3):209-214.

[14] Ampt, A.J., Amoroso, C., et al. Attitudes, norms and controls influencing lifestyle risk factor management in general practice. *BMC Fam Pract* 2009 Aug 26; 10:59. doi: 10.1186/1471-2296-10-59.

[15] Bodenheimer, T., Wagner, E., et al. Improving primary care for patients with chronic illness. *JAMA* 2002 Oct 9; 288(14):1775-1779.

[16] Jordan, J.E., Briggs, A.M. et al. Enhancing patient engagement in chronic disease self-management support initiatives in Australia: the need for an integrated approach. *Med J Aust* 2008 Nov 17; 189(10 Suppl):S9-S13.

[17] Gress, S., Baan, C.A., et al. Co-ordination and management of chronic conditions in Europe: the role of primary care–position paper of the European Forum for Primary Care. *Qual Prim Care* 2009;17(1):75-86.

[18] Haynes, R.B., Ackloo, E., et al. Interventions for enhancing medication adherence. *Cochrane Database Syst Rev* 2008 Apr 16;(2):CD000011. doi: 10.1002/14651858.CD000011.pub3.

[19] Inglis, S., Clark, R., et al. Structured telephone support or telemonitoring programmes for patients with chronic heart failure. *Cochrane Database Syst Rev* 2010 Aug 4;(8):CD007228. doi: 10.1002/14651858.CD007228.pub2.

[20] Minet, L., Moller, S., et al. Mediating the effect of self-care management intervention in type 2 diabetes: a meta-analysis of 47 randomised controlled trials (Structured abstract). *Patient Educ Couns* 2010 Jul; 80(1):29-41. doi: 10.1016/j.pec.2009.09.033. Epub 2009 Nov 10.

[21] Nieuwlaat, R., Wilczynski, N., Navarro, T., Hobson, N., Jeffery, R., Keepanasseril, A., Agoritsas, T., Mistry, N., Lorio, A., Jack, S., Sivaramalingam, B., Iserman, E., Mustafa, R.A., Jedraszewski, D., Cotoi, C., Haynes, R.B. Interventions for enhancing medication adherence (Review). *Cochrane Database Syst Rev* 2014 Nov 20;11:CD000011. doi: 10.1002/14651858.CD000011.pub4.

[22] Battersby, M., Egger, G., Litt, J.C. Self management in lifestyle medicine. In: R.G. Eggers, A. Binns, S. Rossner (Eds.). *Lifestyle Medicine*. Sydney, McGraw-Hill, 2010;48-58.

[23] World Health Organization. Preparing a health care workforce for the 21st century: the challenge of chronic conditions. Geneva, 2005.

[24] Levenstein, J., McCracken, E., et al. The patient-centred clinical method. 1 A model for the doctor-patient interaction in family medicine. *Fam Pract* 1986 Mar; 3(1):24-30.

[25] Weston, R., Brown, J., et al. Patient-centred interviewing Part I: understanding patients' experiences. *Can Fam Physician* 1989 Jan; 35:147-151.

[26] Mead, N., Bower, P. Patient-centredness: a conceptual framework and review of the empirical literature. *Soc Sci Med* 2000 Oct; 51(7):1087-1110.

[27] Stewart, M. Towards a global definition of patient-centred care: the patient should be the judge of patient-centred care. *BMJ* 2001 Feb 24; 322:444-445.

[28] Finset, A. Research on person-centred clinical care. *J Eval Clin Pract 2011;* Apr;17(2): 384-6. doi: 10.1111/j.1365-2753.2010.01608.x. Epub 2011 Jan 5.

[29] Wagner, E., Austin, B., et al. Organising care for patients with chronic illness. *Milbank Q* 1996; 74(4):511-544.

[30] Epstein, R.M., Street, R.L. The values and value of patient-centered care. *Ann Fam Med* 2011 Mar-Apr;9(2):100–103. DOI:10.1370/afm.1239. PMCID: PMC3056855.

[31] Rochfort, A. Patient participation in implementation of quality improvement in general practice. In: Rochfort, A., Kijowska, V., Dubas, K (Eds). Guidebook on Implementation of Quality Improvement in General Practice. European Commission under the Leonardo da Vinci programme, 2012. ISBN 978-83-932788-2-4. Available online: http://ingpinqi.eu/guidebook_EN/index.html [Accessed 2nd March 2016].

[32] Mola, E., De Bonis, J.A., Giancane, R. Integrating patient empowerment as an essential characteristic of the discipline of general practice/family medicine. *Eur J Gen Prac* 2008; 14(2):89-94. doi: 10.1080/13814780802423463.

[33] Grüninger, U., Kissling, B. Die Hausarztmedizin als eigene Disziplin und als Spezialgebiet (Family Medicine –a specialty of its own). *Primary Care* 2005;5(11):269-271.

[34] Barr, V.J., Robinson, S., Marin-Link, B., Underhill, L., Dotts, A., Ravensdale D., Salivaras, S. The expanded chronic care model: an integration of concepts and strategies from population health promotion and the Chronic Care Model. *Hosp Q*. 2003;7(1): 73-82.

[35] Lorig, K.R., Holman, H. Self-management education: history, definition, outcomes, and mechanisms. *Ann Behav Med* 2003 Aug; 26(1):1-7.

[36] Lawn, S., Battersby, M. Capabilities for supporting prevention and chronic condition self-management: a resource for educators of primary health care professionals. Adelaide, Department of Health and Ageing, Australian Government; Flinders University, 2009;39.

[37] Renders, C.M., Valk, G.D., Griffin, S., Wagner, E.H., Eijk, J.T., Assendelft, W.J. Interventions to improve the management of diabetes mellitus in primary care, outpatient and community settings. *Cochrane Database Syst Rev* 2001;(1):CD001481. PMID: 11279717.

[38] Holman, H., Lorig, K. Patient self-management: a key to effectiveness and efficiency in care of chronic disease. *Public Health Rep*2004 May-Jun; 119 (3):239-243.

[39] Muenchberger, H., Kendall, E. Predictors of preventable hospitalization in chronic disease: priorities for change. *J Public Health Policy* 2010 Jul; 31(2):150-63. doi: 10.1057/jphp.2010.3.

[40] Lawn, S., Schoo, A. Supporting self-management of chronic health conditions: common approaches. *Patient Educ Couns* 2010 Aug; 80(2):205-11. doi: 10.1016/j.pec.2009.10.006.

[41] Adams, K., Greiner, A.C., Corrigan, J.M. (Eds). Report of a summit. The first annual crossing the quality chasm summit: A focus on communities. Washington, CD: National Academies Press, 2004.

[42] Johnston, S., Liddy, C., Ives, S.M., Soto E. Literature review on chronic disease self-management. Élisabeth Bruyère Research Institute. Ottawa, Ontario, 2008.

[43] Glasgow, R.E., Davis, C.L., et al. Implementing practical interventions to support chronic illness self-management. *Jt Comm J Qual Saf* 2003 Nov; 29(11):563-574.

[44] Woodcock, A., Kinmonth, A-L. Patient concerns in their first year with type 2 diabetes: patient and practice nurse views. *Patient Educ Couns* 2001 Mar; 42(3):257-270.

[45] Willcox, J., Gill, M. Integrated disease management programs: reflections and learnings from implementation. *Aust J Prim Health* 2007;13(2):113-120. DOI:10.1071/PY07029.

[46] Parlour, R., Slater, P. *An evaluation of the effectiveness of a self-management programme.* Dublin: Health Service Executive, 2011.

[47] Bradley, P.M., Lindsay, B. Care delivery and self-management strategies for adults with epilepsy. *Cochrane Database Syst Rev* 2008; Jan 23;(1):CD006244. doi: 10.1002/14651858.CD006244.pub2.

[48] Deakin, T., McShane, C.E., Cade, J.E., Williams, R.D. Group based training for self-management strategies in people with type 2 diabetes mellitus. *Cochrane Database Syst Rev* 2005 Apr 18; (2):CD003417.

[49] Clark, N., Becker, M.H., Janz, N.K., Lorig, K., Rakowski, W., Anderson, L. Self-management of chronic disease by older adults: a review and questions for research. *J Aging Health*1991 February; 3(1):3-27.

[50] Robinson, L., Newton, J.L., Jones, D., Dawson, P. Promoting self-management and adherence with strength and balance training for older people with long-term conditions: a mixed-methods study. *J Eval Clin Pract* 2014 Aug;20(4):318-26. DOI: 10.1111/jep.12128. Epub 25 April 2014.

[51] McKinstry, B. Do patients wish to be involved in decision making in the consultation. A cross sectional survey with video vignettes. *BMJ* 2000 Oct 7; 321(7265):867-871.

[52] Légaré, F., Ratté, S., et al. Interventions for improving the adoption of shared decision making by healthcare professionals. *Cochrane Database Syst Rev* 2010 May 12; (5):CD006732. DOI: 10.1002/14651858.

[53] Gorter, K.J., Tuytel, G.J., et al. Opinions of patients with type 2 diabetes about responsibility, setting targets and willingness to take medication. A cross-sectional survey. *Patient Educ Couns* 2011 Jul; 84(1):56-61. doi: 10.1016/j.pec.2010.06.019. Epub 2010 Jul 23.

[54] Taggart, J., Chan, B., et al. Patients assessment of chronic illness care (PACIC) in two Australian studies: structure and utility. *J Eval Clin Pract* 2011 Apr; 17(2):215-21. doi: 10.1111/j.1365-2753.2010.01423.x. Epub 2010 Sep 16.

[55] Gensichen, J., Beyer, M., Kuver, C., Wang, H., Gerlach, F.M. [Case management for patients with congestive heart failure under ambulatory care - a critical review,German]. *Z Arztl Forbbild Qualitatssich* 2004 Mar; 98(2):143–154.

[56] Foster, G., Taylor, S.J., et al. Self-management education programmes by lay leaders for people with chronic conditions. *Cochrane Database Syst Rev*2007 Oct 17; (4):CD005108.

[57] Duke, S.A., Colagiuri, S., et al. Individual patient education for people with type 2 diabetes mellitus. *Cochrane Database Syst Rev* 2009 Jan 21; (1):CD005268. doi: 10.1002/14651858.CD005268.pub2.

[58] Peytremann-Bridevaux, I., Gex, G., et al. Chronic disease management programs for adults with asthma (Protocol). *Cochrane Database Syst Rev* 2009; (3):CD007988/DOI: 10.1002/14651858.

[59] Peytremann-Bridevaux, I., Arditi, C., Gex, G., Bridevaux, P.O., Burnand, B. Chronic disease management programmes for adults with asthma. *Cochrane Database Syst Rev*. 2015 May 27; 5:CD007988. doi: 10.1002/14651858.CD007988.pub2.

[60] Gensichen, J., von Korff, M., Rutter, C.M., Seelig, M.D., Ludman, E.J., Lin, E.H.B., Ciechanowski, P., Young, B.A., Wagner, E.H., Katon, W.J. Physician support for diabetes patients and clinical outcomes. *BMC Public Health* 2009 Sep 29; 9:367. doi: 10.1186/1471-2458-9-367.

[61] Bower, P., Kennedy, A., Reeves, D., Rogers, A., Blakeman, T., Chew-Graham, C., Bowen, R., Eden, M., Gardner, C., Hann, M., Lee, V., Morris, R., Protheroe, J., Richardson, G., Sanders, C., Swallow, A., Thompson, D. A cluster randomised controlled trial of the clinical and cost-effectiveness of a 'whole systems' model of self-management support for the management of long- term conditions in primary care: trial protocol. *Implement Sci* 2012 Jan 26; 7:7. doi: 10.1186/1748-5908-7-7.

[62] Phillips, L.S., Brand, W.T., Cook, C.B., Doyle, J.P., El-Kebbi, I.M., Gallina, D.L., Miller, C.D., Ziemer, D.C., Barnes, C.S. Clinical Inertia. *Ann Intern Med* 2001 Nov 6; 135(9):825-834.

[63] Elwyn, G., Frosch, D., Thomson, R., Joseph-Williams, N., Lloyd, A., Kinnersley, P., Cording, E., Tomson. D., Dodd, C., Rollnick, S., Edwards, A., Barry, M. Shared decision making: a model for clinical practice. J Gen Intern Med 2012 Oct; 27(10): 1361-1367. DOI: 10.1007/s11606-012-2077-6.

[64] Kennedy, A., Chew-Graham, C., Blakeman, T., Bowen, A., Gardner, C., Protheroe, J., Rogers, A., Gask, L. Delivering the WISE (Whole Systems Informing Self-Manage-

ment Engagement) training package in primary care: learning from formative evaluation. *Implement Sci* 2010 Jan 29; 5:7. doi: 10.1186/1748-5908-5-7.

[65] Aujoulet, I., d'Hoore, W. Deccache, A. Patient empowerment in theory and practice: polysemy or cacophony? *Patient Educ Couns*. 2007 Apr; 66(1):13-20. Epub 2006 Nov 2.

[66] McAllister, M., Dunn, G., Payne, K., Davies, L., Todd, C. Patient empowerment: the need to consider it as a measurable patient-reported outcome for chronic conditions. *BMC Health Serv Res* 2012 Jun 13; 12::157. PMID: 22694747.

[67] Guadagnoli, E., Ward, P. Patient participation in decision-making. *Soc Sci Med* 1998 Aug; 47(3):329-339.

[68] Anderson, R.M., Funnell, M.M. Patient empowerment: reflections on the challenge of fostering the adoption of a new paradigm. *Patient EducCouns*. 2005 May; 57(2):153-7.

[69] Aujoulat, I., Marcolongo, R., Bonadiman, L., Deccache, A. Reconsidering patient empowerment in chronic illness: a critique of models of self-efficacy and bodily control. *Soc Sci Med* 2008 Mar; 66(5):1228-39. Epub 2007 Dec 21.

[70] Lorig, K., Ritter, P.L., Villa, F.J., Armas, J. Community-based peer-led diabetes self-management: a randomized trial. *Diabetes Educ* 2009 Jul-Aug; 35(4):641-51. doi: 10.1177/0145721709335006. Epub2009 Apr 30.

[71] Funnell, M.M., Anderson, R.M. Patient empowerment: a look back, a look ahead. *Diabetes Educ* 2003 May-Jun; 29(3):454-8, 460, 462 passim.

[72] Anderson, R.M., Funnell, M.M. Patient empowerment: myths and misconceptions. *Patient Educ Couns* 2010 Jun; 79(3):277-282. DOI:10.1016/j.pec.2009.07.025. PMID: 19682830.

[73] Sen, A. Capability and well-being. In: Nussbaum, M.C., Sen, A. (Eds.), The Quality of Life. Oxford, Clarendon Press, 1993.

[74] Anderson, R.M., Funnell, M.M., Fitzgerald, J.T., Marrero, D.G. The diabetes empowerment scale: a measure of psychosocial self-efficacy. *Diabetes Care* 2000 Jun; 23:739-743.

[75] Sibbald, B., Roland, M. Getting research into practice. *J Eval Clin Pract* 1997 Feb; 3(1): 15-21.

[76] Lopez, A., Mathers, C., Ezzati, M., Jamison, D., Murray, C. Measuring the global burden of disease and risk factors, 1990-2001. In: Lopez, A., Mathers, C., Ezzati, M., Jamison, D. Murray, C. (Eds.) *Global Burden of Disease and Risk*.Washington (DC): World Bank; 2006:1-14. Available from: http://www.ncbi.nlm.nih.gov/books/NBK11812/ [Accessed 3rd March 2016].

[77] Holmstrom, I., Roing, M. The relation between patient-centredness and patient empowerment: a discussion of concepts. *Patient EducCouns*. 2010 May; 79(2):167-72. doi: 10.1016/j.pec.2009.08.008. Epub 2009 Sep 11.

[78] EQuiP Working Group on the concept of patient empowerment. Work Package 1c. source: Work Package 1c: EQuiP Working Group on Patient Empowerment for Self-Management in Chronic Conditions. http://www.equip.ch/flx/pecc_we/work_packages/. [Accessed 25 November 2015].

[79] Starfield, B., Shi, L., Macinko, J. Contribution of primary care to health systems and health. *Milbank Q* 2005; 83(3):457-502.

[80] Krist, A.H., Woolf, S.H. A vision for patient-centered health information systems. *JAMA* 2011 Jan 19; 305(3):300-1. doi: 10.1001/jama.2010.2011.

[81] Anderson, R.M. Patient empowerment and the traditional medical model: a case of irreconcilable differences? *Diabetes Care* 1995 Mar; 18(3): 412-5.

[82] Rochfort, A. Patient Empowerment for Patient Self-Management. In: World Book of Family Medicine, European Edition. Wonca, October 2015. http://www.woncaeurope.org/sites/default/files/001%20%E2%80%93%20Patient%20Empowerment_0.pdf. [Accessed 25 November 2015].

Section 2

Integrated Care for Chronic Conditions

Chapter 3

Integrated Care for Heart Failure in Primary Care

Monica Lorenzini, Caterina Ricci, Silvia Riccomi, Federica Abate, Barbara Casalgrandi, Benedetta Quattrini, Gianbattista Spagnoli, Letizia Reggianini and Oreste Capelli

Additional information is available at the end of the chapter

http://dx.doi.org/10.5772/63946

Abstract

Chronic heart failure (CHF or simply HF) is a complex clinical syndrome that involves more than 2% of the general population and over 10% of the older people. For people with reduced ventricular function (the classical HFrEF phenotype), the guideline-directed medical therapy (GDMT) (e.g., Ace-inhibitors, beta-blockers, diuretics, rehabilitation or implantable ventricular devices) demonstrated to be efficacious in reducing hospitalisations and prolonging survival. Vice-versa, the HF with preserved ejection fraction (diastolic HF or HFpEF phenotype) is a much more complex syndrome, in which co-morbidities (such as COPD, depression, anemia, and diabetes, CAD) play a significant role in the decompensation episodes.

As the population ages, the HFpEF phenotype is becoming more frequent and puts more management problems, since the conventional HF therapy is less efficacious in the control of symptoms. A multidisciplinary managed approach, based on the principles of Chronic Care Model, is the most effective tool to ensure best clinical and social outcomes, for both phenotypes. It is critical that every health worker should use counselling tools, such as how to recognise characteristics of the disease or early signs of decompensation and whereby to manage them, the proper use of each drug or how to modify progressing risk factor, to improve the compliance of the patients toward the self-management empowerment.

Finally, we propose a plan of care for patients affected with HF, which allows the integration of multidisciplinary teams and ensures a complete and appropriate management of the cases, in respect of therapeutic responsibility entrusted to the GP.

Keywords: chronic heart failure, preserved ejection fraction, co-morbidities, integrated care, Chronic Care Model

INTECH
open science | open minds

© 2016 The Author(s). Licensee InTech. This chapter is distributed under the terms of the Creative Commons Attribution License (http://creativecommons.org/licenses/by/3.0), which permits unrestricted use, distribution, and reproduction in any medium, provided the original work is properly cited.

1. Introduction

1.1. Chronic heart failure: Definition and diagnosis

Chronic heart failure (CHF or simply HF) is one of the main causes of death and disability in the Western world. It is expected that its presence will continue increasing in the future because of the ageing of the population, the diminution of mortality in the acute phase of coronary heart disease, the increased prevalence of predisposing clinical conditions (diabetes mellitus, arterial hypertension, obesity, etc.), as well as the availability of effective drugs in prolonging the patients' survival. HF in developed countries is mainly a disease of the elderly population: the average age of the patients is in fact 75 years [1].

Continuity of care is one of the basic elements for a correct management of HF, both for its characteristic of chronic disease with more or less frequent exacerbations and for its considerable clinical variability, which manifests itself with different levels of complexity and not uniformly progressive in all stages of its evolution, from the very first symptoms of the terminal stages. This aspect results in a diagnostic difficulty that swings the estimate of prevalence of the disease from 2 to 6.7% of the general population [2, 3].

In fact, as defined in the Report of the American College of Cardiology Foundation/ American Heart Association Task Force on Practice Guidelines 'HF is a complex clinical syndrome that results from any structural or functional impairment of ventricular filling or ejection of blood', but HF should be present as a diastolic dysfunction with a left ventricular ejection fraction (LVEF) greater than 40%. However, some component of diastolic dysfunction is also common in patients with LVEF < 40% [1, 2].

NYHA Class	Level of Clinical Impairment
I	No limitation of physical activity. Ordinary physical activity does not cause undue breathlessness, fatigue, or palpitations.
II	Slight limitation of physical activity. Comfortable at rest, but ordinary physical activity results in undue breathlessness, fatigue, or palpitations.
III	Marked limitation of physical activity. Comfortable at rest, but less than ordinary physical activity results in undue breathlessness, fatigue, or palpitations.
IV	Unable to carry on any physical activity without discomfort. Symptoms at rest can be present. If any physical activity is undertaken, discomfort is increased.

Figure 1. New York Heart Association (NYHA) Heart Failure Symptom Classification System.

The European Task Force on the Diagnosis and Treatment of Acute and Chronic Heart Failure in 2012 stated that: *HF is defined, clinically, as a syndrome in which patients have typical symptoms (e.g. breathlessness, ankle swelling, and fatigue) and signs (e.g. elevated jugular venous pressure, pulmonary crackles, and displaced apex beat) resulting from an abnormality of cardiac structure or function. The diagnosis of HF can be difficult* [4].

On the basis of clinical and structural features of the syndrome, the American College of Cardiology (ACC) and American Heart Association (AHA) developed a four- stage classification of heart failure [5].

Stage A includes patients who are at risk of developing HF but who have no structural heart disease at present. Stage B includes patients with structural heart disease but no symptoms. Stage C includes patients with structural heart disease with current or prior symptomatic heart failure. Stage D includes patients with severe refractory HF. The previous classification of HF, based on the NYHA functional scheme (Figure 1), is used to assess the severity of functional limitations and correlates fairly well with prognosis.

The linkage between ACC/AHA structural staging, NYHA functional classification and community epidemiology (estimated from the Olmsted County Study for people aged more than 45 years) is summarised in Figure 2 [5, 6].

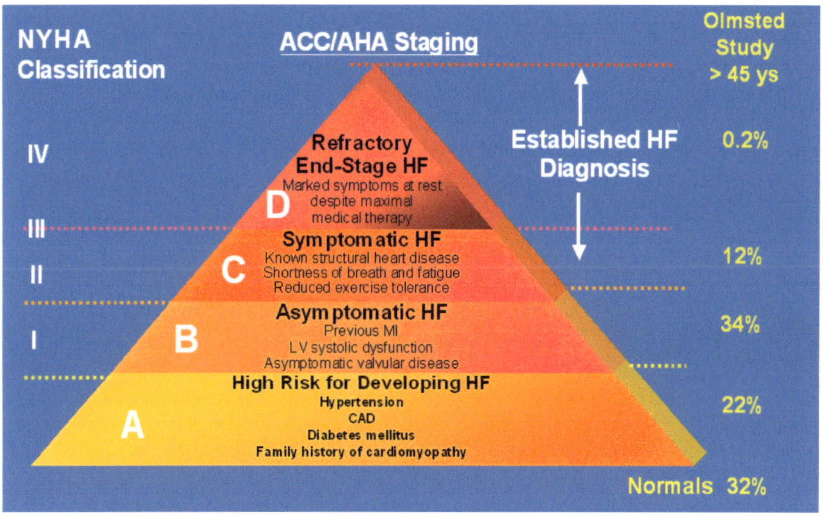

Figure 2. Structural, functional and epidemiologic linkages in CHF (for courtesy of Prof. Tang, Assoc. Prof. of Medicine, Cleveland Clinic Lerner College of Medicine; adapted from [5,6]).

Most patients affected with HF have signs and symptoms of fluid overload and pulmonary congestion, including dyspnea, orthopnea and paroxysmal nocturnal dyspnea. Patients with right ventricular failure have jugular venous distention, peripheral oedema, hepatosplenomegaly and ascites. Others, however, do not have congestive symptoms but have signs and symptoms of low cardiac output, including fatigue, effort intolerance, cachexia and renal hypoperfusion (Table 1).

On physical examination, patients with decompensated heart failure may be tachycardic and tachypneic, with bilateral inspiratory rales, jugular venous distention and oedema. Patients with compensated heart failure will likely have clear lungs but a displaced cardiac apex. Patients with decompensated diastolic dysfunction usually have a loud S4 (which may be palpable), rales and often systemic hypertension.

SYMPTOMS	**SIGNS**
TYPICAL	MORE SPECIFIC
Breathlessness	Elevated jugular venous pressure
Orthopnoea	Hepatojugular reflux
Paroxysmal nocturnal dyspnoea	Third heart sound (gallop rhythm)
Reduced exercise tolerance	Laterally displaced apical impulse
Fatigue, tiredness, increased time to recover after exercise	Cardiac murmur
Ankle swelling	
LESS TYPICAL	LESS SPECIFIC
Nocturnal cough	Peripheral oedema (ankle, sacral, scrotal)
Wheezing	Pulmonary crepitations
Weight gain (>2 kg/week)	Reduced air entry and dullness to percussion at lung bases (pleural effusion)
Weight loss (in advanced heart failure)	Tachycardia
Bloated feeling	Irregular pulse
Loss of appetite	Tachypnoea (>16 breaths/min)
Confusion (especially in the elderly)	Hepatomegaly
Depression	Ascites
Palpitations	Tissue wasting (cachexia)
Syncope	

Table 1. Diagnostic symptoms and signs for chronic heart failure (modified from ESC 2012 [4])

In ambulatory patients suspected of having HF, for an initial working diagnosis and treatment plan, the recommended investigations are [4] **electrocardiogram (ECG), echocardiogram** and some **haematological investigations**:

1. **The ECG** shows the heart rhythm and electrical conduction, i.e. whether there is sinoatrial disease, atrioventricular (AV) block or abnormal intraventricular conduction.

2. **The echocardiogram** provides immediate information on chamber volumes, ventricular systolic and diastolic function, wall thickness and valve function.

3. **Routine biochemical and haematological investigations** are also important, partly to determine whether renin–angiotensin–aldosterone blockade can be initiated safely (renal

http://dx.doi.org/10.5772/63946

function, sodium and potassium) and to exclude anaemia (which can mimic or aggravate HF). Other measurements of blood chemistry, such as calcium, liver enzymes, bilirubin, ferritin and thyroid function, should detect reversible/ treatable causes of HF (e.g. hypocalcaemia, thyroid dysfunction) and co-morbidities (e.g. iron deficiency).

Natriuretic peptide (BNP, NT-proBNP or MR-proANP) dosage and a **chest radiograph (X-ray)** should be useful, but their use for diagnostic purposes is not clearly defined **[4]**.

2. Two phenotypes of chronic HF: reduced or preserved ejection fraction

Most of the evidence supporting interventions in heart failure comes from trials that recruited patients with left ventricular systolic dysfunction (LVSD). However, about 50% of patients with chronic heart failure (CHF) have a preserved ejection fraction (HFpEF), which is especially common in elderly people with highly prevalent co-morbid conditions, and its prevalence is expected to increase over the next decades [7, 8].

The necessary criteria for diagnosing heart failure with reduced ejection fraction (HF-rEF) or preserved ejection fraction (HF- pEF or diastolic heart failure) are reported in Table 2. Echo-cardiographic evaluation is essential to differentiate the structural abnormalities of the two phenotypes: HFpEF is usually defined as an ejection fraction equal to or greater than 50%, while the reduced ejection fraction phenotype (HF-rEF) has an LVEF less than 40%. Both ESC and ACC/AHA guidelines define a mild left ventricular systolic dysfunction (for EF 35–50%) that probably represents another phenotype in HF spectrum [8, 9].

Therapies that improve outcome in people with HFrEF have not been found to help people with HFpEF, further supporting the idea that these two kinds of HF are fundamentally different [9].

The diagnosis of **HF-rEF (reduced ejection fraction)** requires **three** conditions to be satisfied:	The diagnosis of **HF-pEF (preserved ejection fraction)** requires **four** conditions to be satisfied:
1. Symptoms typical of HF	1. Symptoms typical of HF
2. Signs typical of HF (may not be present in the early stages and patients treated with diuretics)	2. Signs typical of HF (especially in HF-pEF they may not be present in the early stages and patients treated with diuretics)
3. Reduced left ventricular ejection fraction (LVEF): < 40%	3. Normal or only mildly reduced LVEF (35–50%) and left ventricule not dilated
	4. Relevant structural heart disease (left ventricular hypertrophy/left atrial enlargement) and/or diastolic dysfunction

Table 2. Criteria for diagnosing and differentiate CHF phenotypes (modified from ESC 2012 [4])

Exercise intolerance is the principal clinical feature in HFpEF. People complain of debilitating symptoms: the elevation of filling pressures during even modest exercise causes significant dyspnea and fatigue [7, 9]. NICE guidelines recommend the implementation of exercise training in HFpEF, but the evidence only evaluates surrogate endpoints such as exercise capacity and quality of life [10].

3. The guideline-directed medical therapy (GDMT) for chronic heart failure

The treatments for heart failure become progressively more complex, gradually the clinical picture worsens (Figure 3) [11]. However, there is a high overall annual mortality (up to 20%), both for HFrEF or HFpEF [12] particularly in patients with higher NYHA Classes symptoms [13].

General measures, such as the attention to diet and good lifestyle, weight monitoring, patient education and close medical follow-up, should be done on all patients, while medical therapy is based on progressive staging and symptoms classification [13].

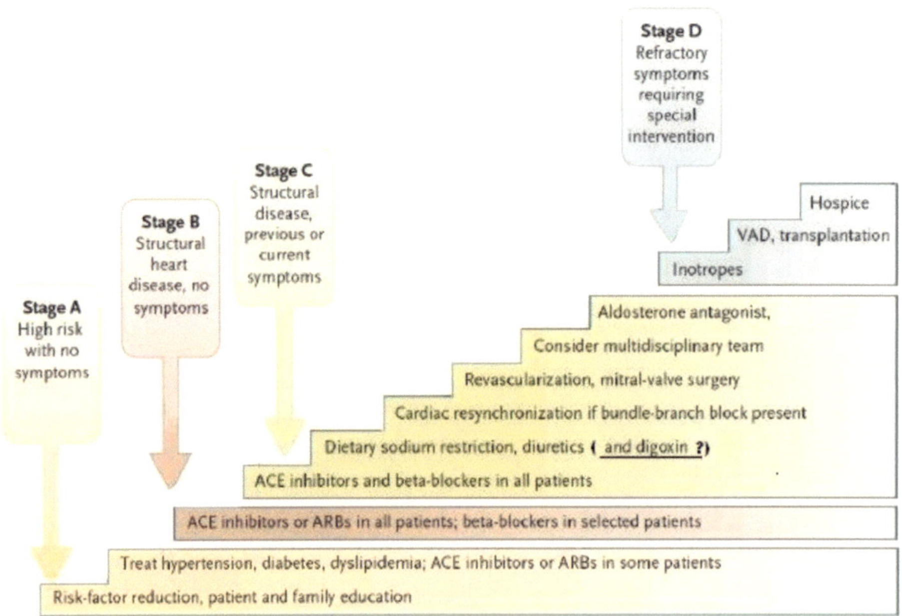

Figure 3. The progression and complexity of treatments for HF (Modified from [11]).

The term guideline-directed medical therapy (GDMT) has been conjugated by the ACCF/AHA Task Force on Practice Guidelines to represent optimal medical therapy as defined by ACCF/

http://dx.doi.org/10.5772/63946

AHA guideline recommended therapies (primarily Class I evidence) [1]. The GDMT for patients with CHF is resumed in Figure 4 [13].

Even if the recommendations for the use of drugs in HF derived principally from studies that recruited patients with left ventricular systolic dysfunction (LVSD) (HFrEF), treatments with same principles are also useful for patients with HFpEF and relevant cardiovascular co-morbidities, such as hypertension and coronary artery disease (CAD).

Unfortunately, trials using the same medications employed for the treatment of HFrEF have not shown any significant improvements on survival [8, 12].

ACC/AHA Stage	B	C		D
NYHA Classification	I	II – III		IV
Symptoms[a] / Treatments	Asymptomatic	Symptoms, Current or Prior		Recurrent or Ongoing Rest Dyspnea
		Never Hospitalized	History of Hospitalization	
ACEI	Yes	Yes	Yes	Yes
Beta blocker (BBs)	Yes[a]	Yes	Yes	Yes[b]
Aldosterone antagonist		Yes	Yes	Yes
Isosorbide dinitrate-hydralazine		Selected patients[c]	Selected patients[c]	Selected patients[c]
Diuretic		If congestion PRN	If congestion PRN	Yes
ARB		PRN[d]	PRN[d]	PRN[d]
Digoxin		PRN[d]	PRN[d]	PRN[d]
Consider AICD/ Bi-V pacemaker	Selected patients[e]	Yes	Yes	Yes

Abbreviations: **ACEI: Angiotensin converting enzyme inhibitor ARB: Angiotensin receptor blocker**
PRN: as needed **AICD: Automatic Implantable Cardioverter Defibrillator**

Green: Recommended | **Orange: To be considered.**

Notes:

[a] No explicit evidence of benefit exists for BBs among asymptomatic patients, although many patients in this class will have other indications for BBs, such as coronary artery disease (CAD).

[b] BBs may be continued safely for patients with rest dyspnea except in patients with signs of congestion or hemodynamic instability.

[c] The combination of isosorbide dinitrate and hydralazine benefited patients self-reported as African American. This combination may be added for patients who remain symptomatic despite therapy with ACEIs and BBs and as tolerated without reducing the doses of ACEI or BBs to subtarget doses.

[d] These interventions may provide symptomatic benefit. If no benefit is perceived, the medications may be withdrawn. In the case of digoxin, however, withdrawal may lead to clinical deterioration and should be done with caution. Little evidence exists to support the safety of ACEI/aldosterone antagonists/ARBs in the same patient. All these agents can increase potassium levels.

[e] Indication only for asymptomatic patients with ischemic cardiomyopathy.

Figure 4. GDMT for patients with HFrEF (adapted from [13], with permission).

The only indication to the use of diuretics in chronic HFpEF is for symptomatic relief of acute or chronic congestion (see Figure 3). The doses of diuretics should be adjusted continuously, especially when the patient achieves euvolaemia, as further diuresis and dehydration may decrease preload and cardiac output [8].

The role of the multidisciplinary team in the continuing management of heart failure patients is pivotal and all the principal guidelines on HF management underline that the complexity of both the diagnostic process and the therapeutic options, as well as the continuing difficulties in the diagnosis and management of HFpEF, dictate the recurrent involvement of specialists [1, 4, 5, 10, 14].

4. Rehabilitation for patients with chronic heart failure

A rehabilitation program has three main components: education, counselling and exercise [10]. Education and counselling are usually incorporated into standard care (see below), while the role of exercise-based rehabilitation programs in the management of patients with HF is not completely defined. There is some evidence that cardiac rehabilitation can be useful to improve functional capacity, exercise duration, health-related quality of life and mortality [1, 4], particularly in patients with HFrEF [15]. Despite the paucity of direct evidence in HFpEF, recommendations for rehabilitation should relate to all patients with heart failure without contraindications, since symptoms and prognosis of patients with HFpEF do not differ significantly from those with heart failure due to LVSD [7, 10]. A program of rehabilitation should include patients with symptomatic heart failure, NYHA class II–III, without limitations for age or sex. A psychological and educational component in the program would assure better results of the intervention [10].

The optimum exercise 'prescription' is uncertain: it ranges from walking to intensive gym-based activity including resistance and aerobic exercises and exercises within the swimming pool [4, 10]. In the absence of specific programs for patients with HF, they can also be enrolled in rehabilitation within other existing cardiac rehabilitation programs (i.e. post-myocardial infarction and post-cardiac surgery [10]).

Healthcare-based rehabilitation programs are likely to be cost-effective in different populations and for different healthcare systems [16].

5. Integrated care for heart failure: The Chronic Care Model

In 2009 Jencks et al [17] demonstrated that heart failure is the most frequent cause of rehospitalisation in Medicare: about 27% of patients discharged with HF were re-admitted within 30 days. The majority of them did not receive a visit from a doctor in the period they stay at home, after discharge. Discharge planning (i.e. an individualised plan for a patient before the patient leaves hospital to home) combined with additional post-discharge support can reduce unplanned readmission to hospital for patients with congestive heart failure [18, 19].

http://dx.doi.org/10.5772/63946

Evidence suggests that systems of care for patients with HF improve adherence to published guidelines and clinical outcomes if involve collaborative care with specialists, multidisciplinary teams (including primary care), with a focus on transitions of care and chronic disease management [19–23].

All the guidelines on HF management recommend a coordinating care along the continuum of HF and throughout the chain-of-care delivered by the various services, within the healthcare system [1, 4, 10, 14]. The natural setting to develop this coordination of care is the Chronic Care Model (CCM), developed by Wagner and colleagues at the end of the nineties, 'to bridge the gap and translate knowledge between evidence-based chronic disease care and actual care practices' [24]. The framework, which is centred in primary care, posits six interrelated elements that are key to high quality chronic disease care: self-management support, redesigning delivery systems, decision support that is system wide, clinical information technology, linkages to community resources and health care system organisation [24].

Recently, the National Heart Foundation of Australia published guidance on policy and system changes to improve the quality of care for people with chronic heart failure (CHF). The recommendations point to reduce emergency presentations, hospitalisations and premature death among patients with CHF [14]. Among the most critical points to overcome there are:

- To ensure equity of access for everyone in disadvantaged areas, including the most vulnerable people in socio-economic frailty and the cultural minorities.
- Lack of data and inadequate identification of people with CHF: this leads to ineffectiveness in measuring outcomes and evaluating the CHF care provided. The development of mechanisms to promote data linkage across care transitions is essential.
- The enhanced community-based management of CHF, across the empowerment of general practitioners to lead care.
- Future research activity needs to ensure the translation of valuable knowledge and high-quality evidence into practice.

The practical application of these principles is included in the recommendation n. 10.2 from ACCF/AHA guidelines [1]: *Every patient with HF should have a clear, detailed, and evidence-based plan of care that ensures the achievement of GDMT goals, effective management of co-morbid conditions, timely follow-up with the healthcare team, appropriate dietary and physical activities, and compliance with secondary prevention guidelines for cardiovascular disease. This plan of care should be updated regularly and made readily available to all members of each patient's healthcare team.*

A management program for patients with HF (both with reduced and preserved ejection fraction) needs particular characteristics and components (Figure 5) [4].

Primary care plays a central role in the early identification of HF, transitions to and from acute care settings, self-care promotion, managing co-morbidities and end-of-life care [23, 25]. However, a recent systematic review of 22 studies has pointed out barriers and facilitators of implementing the chronic care model in primary care. The inner setting of the organisation, the process of implementation and characteristics of the individual healthcare providers are

Characteristics	1. Based on a multidisciplinary approach (cardiologists, primary care physicians, nurses, pharmacists, etc.) 2. Targeted to high-risk symptomatic patients 3. Including competent and professionally educated staff
Components	• Optimized medical and device management • Adequate patient education, with special emphasis on adherence and self-care • Patient involvement in symptom monitoring and flexible diuretic use • Follow-up after discharge (regular clinic and/or home-based visits; possibly telephone support or remote monitoring) • Increased access to healthcare (through in-person follow-up and by telephone contact; possibly through remote monitoring) • Facilitated access to care during episodes of decompensation • Assessment of (and appropriate intervention in response to) an unexplained increase in weight, nutritional status, functional status, quality of life, and laboratory findings • Access to advanced treatment options • Provision of psychosocial support to patients and family and/or caregivers

Figure 5. Management programmes for patients with HF rEF and HFpEF: essential characteristics and components (adapted from [4]).

the major emerging themes. The importance of assessing organisational capacity and needs is crucial prior to and during the implementation of the CCM, as well as gaining a better understanding of health care providers and organisational perspective [26].

6. Management of co-morbidities

Frailty and multiple co-morbidities contribute to non-compliance, leading to higher rate of hospitalisation, rehospitalisation, and ultimately institutionalisation and death [27].

Co-morbidities are important in patients with HF for four main reasons [4]:

1. They may affect the use of some drugs for HF (e.g. in some patients with renal dysfunction the use of renin–angiotensin system inhibitors may be discouraged);
2. Some drugs, useful for co-morbidities symptoms, may decompensate HF (e.g. NSAIDs for pain in arthritis);
3. The drugs for different conditions may interact and reduce patient compliance to treatments: e.g. beta-blockers for HF and beta-agonists for obstructive pulmonary disease;
4. Most co-morbidities are associated with worse clinical status and are predictors of poor prognosis in HF (e.g. diabetes). Some co-morbidities become subject to treatment (e.g. anemia) to improve HF.

Management of co-morbidities is particularly critical in HF patients with preserved ejection fraction (the so-called diastolic heart failure or HFpEF) who are older and often affected with multimorbidity. Patients with HFpEF should be managed with an integrated approach by their clinical features, addressing underlying co-morbidities known to cause or exacerbate HF [28]. Predisposing and precipitating factors for patients with HFpEF are reported in Table 3.

PREDISPOSING FACTORS	PRECIPITATING FACTORS
Advanced age	Recurrent ischemia
Female sex	Atrial fibrillation
Obesity	Renal failure
Hypertension	Sepsis
Diabetes	
Coronary artery disease	

Table 3. Predisposing and precipitating factors for HFpEF in older [28]

Other significant co-morbidities are anemia, COPD, depression, cachexia, gout, and hyperlipidemia [4]. Cardiovascular deaths constitute the majority of deaths in both HFpEF and HFrEF. However, the proportion of total deaths that are cardiovascular related is higher in HFrEF than in HFpEF. Conversely, non-cardiovascular deaths constitute a larger proportion of deaths in HFpEF than in HFrEF [12].

7. Counselling and patient's empowerment

In chronic illness, patient- centred care (PCC) has a beneficial effect on healthcare professional-patient concordance regarding treatment plans, patient health outcomes and patient satisfaction and respects patients' desired level of involvement in healthcare decisions [30]. Patient education is focused on the patient's knowledge about his pathology in making the right choices about his/her health and not just decisions about the disease, how the disease affects his/her role in working life, couple or community life [31]. Counselling is the better professional activity to guide, support and develop the self-management and empowerment both of the patient and his/her caregiver(s), promoting knowledge and skills to self-care, and stimulating the ability to make self-choices.

The self-management of chronic disease is essential for optimising health outcomes [32–34]. A patient-centred approach for CHF management is widely recommended [4,10, 29].

Counselling for CHF management should be focused on simple actions that the patient and / or the caregiver should practice Table 4.

A. Characteristics of disease	Explain the origin of symptoms;
B. How to identify early signs of decompensation and what to do with them	Identify specific signs and symptoms such as increasing fatigue, worsening dyspnea, appearance of edema; Daily weight and how to proceed in case of significant increase: contact details of the care manager, variation of the diet , fluid intake and diuretics;
C. Instructions on the proper use of each drug	Explain the rationale for each drug, adverse effects and possible consequences of a missed dose. Repeat the treatment pattern;
D. Modify risk factors progressing	Smoking cessation, glycemic, blood pressure and weight control, motor activity, alcohol intake;
E. Importance of therapeutic adherence	Detect and try to solve any obstacle to the compliance with drug therapy and lifestyle.

Table 4. Counselling for CHF management: what it is basic for patient and caregiver

8. Integrated care for HF in Italy: a clinical pathway implementation

Patients suffering from HF exhibit different clinic characteristics and care needs depending on the stage of the disease [5, 11]. The effective management of this disease should be related to a territorial- and hospital- integrated approach, adapted to the needs of the individual patient [13, 30, 35, 36].

If the clinical condition is stable, the patient should be followed on an outpatient basis with the integrated involvement of general practitioners (GPs), nurses and specialists [20, 22, 23, 37–41]. In advanced stages, a more intensive support like the hospital one and/or integrated home it might be necessary [42–48].

As reported by Vedel and Khanassov [18], transitional care interventions (TCIs) and high intensity- integrated management models significantly reduce risks of rehospitalisation and emergency department visits. A long duration (more than 6 months) involvement of GPs, nurses, and cardiologists is better than a shorter one.

We propose an integrated management care for patients affected with HF, which is based on the recommendations of the European Society of Cardiology [4]. This model allows the integration of multidisciplinary teams, ensuring a complete and appropriate management of the cases, in respect of therapeutic responsibility entrusted to the GP. For each stage of the ACC/AHA classification [1], functions, activities and tasks of each professional are identified. In stage A (Table 5) and D (Table 6) the professionals involved, despite being the same, often operate with different levels of integration, while the real multiprofessional integration occurs in stages B and C. For this reason the latter are presented in comparison (Table 7).

Finally, in Table 8, a synoptic planning of different programmed activity is reported.

http://dx.doi.org/10.5772/63946

STAGE A	
	According to the ACC/AHA classification, patients in stage A are those at risk of developing a structural heart disease for the presence of cardiovascular risk factors or particular clinical situations, such as:
	• Hypertension • Multi system atherosclerosis • Diabetes mellitus • Metabolic syndrome or obesity • Chronic renal failure • Prolonged intake of cardiotoxic drugs • Familiarity of cardiomyopathy
	Role and tasks of the professionals
	• *GP:*
	◦ Identification of patients with risk factors (e.g. hypertension , diabetes, dyslipidemia, obesity, sedentary) ◦ Non-pharmacological control of risk factors (e.g. promoting physical activity, weight control, alcohol consumption) ◦ Setting and titration of personalised drug therapy ◦ Clinical and instrumental follow-up
	• ***Nurses:***
	◦ Group health education for patients and their families, in particular oriented to the promotion of healthy lifestyles, proper nutrition and to the adherence of pharmacological and non-pharmacological therapeutic prescription
	• ***Specialists:***
	◦ Counselling for patients with problems inadequately controlled by first-level interventions

Table 5. Integrated activities on HF stage A, divided for different professional tasks

STAGE D	
	Stage D is characterised by patients suffering from HF with frequent exacerbations despite maximal medical therapy, which may require, in highly selected cases, specialised treatments such as mechanical support to the circulation, fluid removal procedures, continuous inotropic infusions and heart transplant. In most cases, however, the patient benefits from a palliative care program (integrated home assistance, hospice).
	Roles and tasks of the professionals
	• *GP:*
	◦ Request of hospitalisation when indicated ◦ Adjustment of drug therapy based on therapeutic needs of individual patient ◦ Clinical and instrumental follow-up based on the clinical

	characteristics of the individual patient, in agreement with the specialist ◦ Early diagnosis of aggravations of heart failure conditions with identification of precipitating factors ◦ Evaluation and control of co-morbidities ◦ Activation of integrated home care services and access to patient's home
	• *Nurses:*
STAGE D	◦ Periodic evaluation of the parameters (e.g. blood pressure, cardiac frequency and body weight) ◦ Individual health education of the patient and his family, in particular verification of patient's adherence and persistence to the therapeutic drug prescription, lifestyle and to the correct alimentation ◦ Periodic telephone contact (from half-yearly to weekly) for information on taking the drugs, patient's subjective symptoms, ability to perform daily activities, changes in the quality of sleep, changes in body weight, onset of intercurrent diseases ◦ Ambulatory monitoring (from half-yearly to monthly) or periodic home (from monthly to weekly) for the relief of the parameters completed by the judgement of the specialist/GP on patient's condition ◦ Nursing interventions on related symptoms based on the personalised care plan
	• *Specialists:*
	◦ Request of hospitalisation when indicated ◦ Recognition of aggravation of heart failure conditions with identification of precipitating factors ◦ Adjustment of drug therapy based on therapeutic needs of individual patient ◦ Clinical and instrumental follow-up based on the clinical characteristics of the individual patient, in agreement with GP ◦ Intervention in case of clinical worsening without prompt response to therapy or any complications ◦ Indication for AICD (automatic implantable cardioverter defibrillator) ◦ Indication to ultrafiltration ◦ Home access on request of the GP

Table 6. Integrated activities on HF stage D, divided for different professional tasks

http://dx.doi.org/10.5772/63946

Professionals	STAGE B	STAGE C
GP	• Identification of patients with stage B: ▪ Echocardiographic diagnosis of structural heart disease that does not present and have not applied in the past signs and symptoms of HF; ▪ patient with previous myocardial infarction; ▪ patient with valvular heart disease at least moderate; • setting and adjustment of personalised drug therapy, personalised clinical and instrumental follow up, according to the specialist, • Transmission of the names at the computerised archive.	• clinical evaluation and request of medical instrumental/laboratory examinations of I level in presence of signs/symptoms of HF; • specialist referral for diagnostic confirmation; hospitalisation when indicated; • first etiological identification and prognostic stratification; • activation of integrated care program and transmission of patient names in the computer archive; • setting and / or adjustment of the therapy; • personalised clinical and instrumental follow up; • early detection of exacerbations and diagnosis of precipitants factors.
Nurse	• health education (patient/family) oriented to the promotion of healthy lifestyles and nutrition and pharmacological and non-pharmacological therapeutic adherence; • education of the patient to the self-control of arterial pressure parameters, cardiac frequency, body weight; • periodic evaluation of clinical and care parameters; • reporting to the general practitioner (GP) of the patient with relevant issues and collaboration for the diagnostic and therapeutic management; • opening and updating the computerised clinic folder. In this stage other resources can be activated (e.g. anti-smoking centres, gyms safe) in order to better control the risk factors.	• health education (patient/family), in particular pharmacological and non-pharmacological therapeutic adherence; • periodic evaluation of clinical parameters such as arterial pressure, cardiac frequency, body weight; • monitoring of the patient by phone contact (from half-year to weekly or as needed – for evaluation therapy compliance, symptoms, weight, intercurrent diseases); • ambulatory monitoring (from semi-annual to monthly or as needed) or periodic home visits (from monthly to weekly); • point of reference for the patient (it is specified that in the role of disease manager, the nurse becomes a reference for the patient for issues related to pathology).
Cardiologist/ internist	• diagnostic/therapeutic confirmation of structural heart disease; • setting of clinical and instrumental follow-up, in agreement with the GP; consulting for issues not adequately controlled by the first level interventions; • indication for hospitalisation for	• clinical, instrumental (echocardiography) and laboratory evaluation for confirmation/exclusion of the diagnosis of HF; • etiological identification of precipitating/favouring factors and prognostic stratification;

Professionals	STAGE B	STAGE C
	screening of the causes of myocardial damage/evaluation of any indications in non-pharmacological strategies (revascularisation, correction of valve disorders, device implant); • each surgery should have a reference specialist/ambulatory; • if the patient has a different reference doctor, the GP is responsible to verify that inspections are carried out with similar cadences to those of the structured path.	• custom setting and / or adjusting drug therapy; clinical and personal instrumental follow up in collaboration with the GP; • programming non-pharmacological therapeutic procedures (e.g. implantable devices, such as AICD, CRT-P, CRT-D); • intervention in case of clinical worsening without prompt response to therapy or to the appearance of complications.

Table 7. Integrated activities on HF stages B and C, divided for different professional tasks

Stage ACC/AHA and NYHA grading	Care's goals	Action	At least X times/ year follow –up*			Notes
			3	2	1	
STAGE A	Hypertension treatment, smoking cessation, dyslepidemia treatment, promoting regular physical exercise, abolition of alcohol and drugs, metabolic syndrome control	GP visit				Unplanned evaluation
		Nursing assessment				Unplanned evaluation
		ECG+ specialistic visit				Unplanned evaluation
		Echocardiogram				As needed (hypertension and/or diabetes and/or chronic renal failure with signs of organ damage) to each chemotherapy cycle (in patients receiving cardiotoxic drugs) every 3–5 years in case of family history of cardiomyopathy
STAGE B	As stage A + pharmacological therapy of the structural heart disease, non -pharmacological therapy, if indicated (revascularisation, AICD, correction of valvulopathy)	GP visit		x		And as needed
		Nursing assessment		x		Evaluation in alternation at GP
		ECG+ specialistic visit			x	And as needed
		Echocardiogram				Every 2 years/as needed (if clinic modifications/ exacerbations)
STAGE C NYHA I–II	As stages A + B + reducing salt intake, heart failure therapy, implantable devices	GP visit	x			And as needed

Stage ACC/AHA and NYHA grading	Care's goals	Action	At least X times/ year follow –up* 3	2	1	Notes
		Nursing assessment	x			Monitoring of clinical parameters (blood pressure, cardiac frequency, weight) in alternance with GP
	(such as AICD, CRT-P, CRT-D) when indicated	ECG+ specialistic visit			x	And as needed
		Echocardiogram				As needed (if clinic modifications/ exacerbations)
		Blood tests (blood count, creatinine, Na +/K+, glycemia, transaminases)			x	Other surveys according to research
		GP visit	x			And as needed
		Nursing assessment	x			Quarterly monitoring of clinical parameters (blood pressure, cardiac frequency, weight) in alternance with GP
STAGE C NYHA III	As A and B + reducing salt intake, heart failure therapy, implantable devices (such as AICD, CRT-P, CRT-D) when indicated	ECG+ specialistic visit		x		
		Echocardiogram				As needed (if clinic modifications/exacerbation)
		Blood tests (blood count, creatinine, Na +/K+, glycemia, transaminases)			x	Other surveys according to research
STAGE D (Home visits)	Palliative care program or transplantation program					

*The follow-up planning should consider the following variables: NYHA class, clinical and therapeutic instability, repeated hospital admissions, echocardiographic features and exam values.

Table 8. Managed planning for integrated assistance in all HF stages

9. Conclusions

To be effective, an integrated assistance program for the patient with heart failure needs the continuous cooperation of the multidisciplinary team. Integrated care programs have definitively demonstrated a significant reduction in mortality, hospital admissions and readmissions, as well as visits to the emergency department [49].

However, lack of communication between hospital and primary care seems to be the principal critical issue in the continuity of care, both for hospital discharge or for the specialist outpatient report [18, 37].

The general practitioner (GP), with the nurses' collaboration, should manage patients with stable conditions with periodical checks focused on the active involvement of the patient, the constant adaptation of the therapy, the verification of clinical stability, the early detection of worsening of the disease and its causes.

Following every consultation, the health professional should check the patient's understanding of what they have been told. They should ask patients with similar questions: *To be sure that I have explained everything correctly, could you explain to me how you will take your medication?* or *Can you tell me what you found most important from our conversation?* The patients should be able to explain or demonstrate, using their words, what has just been discussed with them [50].

In patients with advanced disease, the specialist monitoring must be flexible, and the consultation should provide clear indications, preferably written, to the patient and family members on when to request the intervention of GP and on signs/symptoms of destabilisation that require specialist advice (Table 9).

Information sending by the GP (patient's summary)	**Specialist outpatient report**
• Current therapy regimen	• Objectivity at visit time and disease stability
• Patient's compliance level	• Stratification of the risk of events after instrumental tests
• Adverse drug events (if any)	• Prescribed treatment with any eventual change compared with the previous treatment and Indications for drug titration
• Major recent intercurrent events, also about co-morbidities	• Evaluation of the presence of co-morbidity about instrumental/ laboratory outcomes
• Results of blood tests (e.g. renal function monitoring)	• Program of specialistic follow-up and indications of instrumental/ laboratory controls
	• Indication and contents of specific training activities directed to the patient and caregiver(s), about the disease, therapy set, and principles of self-management
	• Preferential telephone contacts to communicate with the centre for acute problems

Table 9. Fundamental aspects of the communication between specialist/general practitioner (GP) in the follow-up of patients with heart failure

http://dx.doi.org/10.5772/63946

To standardise multidisciplinary dialogue and assess the effectiveness of clinical pathway, the local health authorities should organise recurrent multiprofessional audit on data collected locally and training on path troubles and care results.

A challenge for the future assistance to the patient with heart failure would be the diagnosis and management of the HF with preserved ejection fraction (HFpEF). As a matter of fact, HFpEF is predicted to be the dominant phenotype of heart failure in the next decade, and the principal intervention is to identify and treat risk factors and co-morbidities associated, first of all, arterial hypertension.

Author details

Monica Lorenzini[1], Caterina Ricci[1], Silvia Riccomi[1], Federica Abate[2], Barbara Casalgrandi[2], Benedetta Quattrini[2], Gianbattista Spagnoli[3], Letizia Reggianini[4] and Oreste Capelli[1*]

*Address all correspondence to: o.capelli@ausl.mo.it

1 Primary Health Care Department, Local Health Authority of Modena, Italy

2 Clinical Governance, Local Health Authority of Modena, Italy

3 Health Director, Local Health Authority of Modena, Italy

4 Heart Failure Clinic, University of Modena and Reggio Emilia, Italy

References

[1] Yancy CW, Jessup M, Bozkurt B, Butler J, Casey DE Jr, Drazner MH, Fonarow GC, Geraci SA, Horwich T, Januzzi JL, Johnson MR, Kasper EK, Levy WC, Masoudi FA, McBride PE, McMurray JJ, Mitchell JE, Peterson PN, Riegel B, Sam F, Stevenson LW, Tang WH, Tsai EJ, Wilkoff BL. (2013): American College of Cardiology Foundation; American Heart Association Task Force on Practice Guidelines. 2013 ACCF/AHA guideline for the management of heart failure: a report of the American College of Cardiology Foundation/American Heart Association Task Force on Practice Guidelines. J Am Coll Cardiol. 62(16):e147-239. Epub 2013 Jun 5.

[2] Owan TE, Hodge DO, Herges RM, Jacobsen SJ, Roger VL, Redfield MM. (2006): Trends in prevalence and outcome of heart failure with preserved ejection fraction. N Engl J Med. 355(3):251-9.

[3] Roger VL. (2013): Epidemiology of heart failure. Circ Res. 113(6):646-59. Review.

[4] McMurray JJ, Adamopoulos S, Anker SD, Auricchio A, Böhm M, Dickstein K, Falk V, Filippatos G, Fonseca C, Gomez-Sanchez MA, Jaarsma T, Køber L, Lip GY, Maggioni

AP, Parkhomenko A, Pieske BM, Popescu BA, Rønnevik PK, Rutten FH, Schwitter J, Seferovic P, Stepinska J, Trindade PT, Voors AA, Zannad F, Zeiher A; ESC Committee for Practice Guidelines. (2012): ESC guidelines for the diagnosis and treatment of acute and chronic heart failure. Developed in collaboration with the Heart Failure Association (HFA) of the ESC. Eur Heart J. 33(14):1787-847. Epub 2012 May 19. Erratum in: Eur Heart J. 2013 Jan;34(2):158.

[5] Jessup M, Abraham WT, Casey DE, Feldman AM, Francis GS, Ganiats TG, Konstam MA, Mancini DM, Rahko PS, Silver MA, Stevenson LW, Yancy CW, writing on behalf of the 2005 Guideline Update for the Diagnosis and Management of Chronic Heart Failure in the Adult Writing Committee. (2009): Focused update: ACCF/AHA guidelines for the diagnosis and management of heart failure in adults: a report of the American College of Cardiology Foundation/American Heart Association Task Force on Practice Guidelines. Circulation. 119:1977-2016.

[6] Ammar KA, Jacobsen SJ, Mahoney DW, Kors JA, Redfield MM, Burnett JC Jr, Rodeheffer RJ. (2007): Prevalence and prognostic significance of heart failure stages: application of the American College of Cardiology/American Heart Association heart failure staging criteria in the community. Circulation. 115(12):1563-70. Epub 2007 Mar 12.

[7] Palau P, Núñez E, Domínguez E, Sanchis J, Núñez J. (2016): Physical therapy in heart failure with preserved ejection fraction: a systematic review. Eur J Prev Cardiol. 23(1):4-13. Epub 2014 Dec 8.Review.

[8] Irizarry Pagán EE, Vargas PE, López-Candales A. (2016): The clinical dilemma of heart failure with preserved ejection fraction: an update on pathophysiology and management for physicians. Postgrad Med J. pii: postgradmedj-2015-133859.

[9] Borlaug BA. (2016): Defining HFpEF: where do we draw the line? Eur Heart J. 37(5): 463-5. doi: 10.1093/eurheartj/ehv561. Epub 2015 Nov 3.

[10] National Clinical Guideline Centre (UK). (2010): Chronic Heart Failure: National Clinical Guideline for Diagnosis and Management in Primary and Secondary Care: Partial Update [Internet]. London: Royal College of Physicians (UK); Aug. http://www.nice.org.uk/nicemedia/live/13099/50517/50517.pdf.

[11] Jessup M, Brozena S. (2003): Heart failure. N Engl J Med. 348(20):2007-18. Review.

[12] Chan MM, Lam CS. (2013): How do patients with heart failure with preserved ejection fraction die? Eur J Heart Fail. 15(6):604-13. Epub 2013 Apr 21. Review.

[13] Nicklas JM, Bleske BE, Van Harrison R, Hogikyan RV, Kwok Y, Chavey WE. (2013): Heart failure: clinical problem and management issues. Prim Care. 40(1):17-42. Review.

[14] Page K, Marwick TH, Lee R, Grenfell R, Abhayaratna WP, Aggarwal A, Briffa TG, Cameron J, Davidson PM, Driscoll A, Garton-Smith J, Gascard DJ, Hickey A, Korczyk D, Mitchell JA, Sanders R, Spicer D, Stewart S, Wade V. (2014): National Heart

Foundation of Australia. A systematic approach to chronic heart failure care: a consensus statement. Med J Aust. 201(3):146-50.

[15] Taylor RS, Sagar VA, Davies EJ, et al. (2014) : Exercise-based rehabilitation for heart failure. Cochrane Database Syst Rev. 4: CD003331.

[16] Hagberg LA, Lindholm L. (2006): Cost-effectiveness of healthcare-based interventions aimed at improving physical activity. Scand J Public Health. 34(6):641-53.

[17] Jencks SF, Williams MV, Coleman EA. (2009): Rehospitalizations among patients in the Medicare fee-for-service program. N Engl J Med. 360(14):1418-28. Erratum in: N Engl J Med. 2011 Apr 21;364(16):1582.

[18] Vedel I, Khanassov V. (2015): Transitional care for patients with congestive heart failure: a systematic review and meta-analysis. Ann Fam Med. 13(6):562-71. Review.

[19] Gonçalves-Bradley DC, Lannin NA, Clemson LM, Cameron ID, Shepperd S. (2016): Discharge planning from hospital. Cochrane Database Syst Rev. 1:CD000313. Review.

[20] Zwarenstein M1, Goldman J, Reeves S. (2009): Interprofessional collaboration: effects of practice-based interventions on professional practice and healthcare outcomes. Cochrane Database Syst Rev. (3):CD000072. doi: 10.1002/14651858.CD000072.pub2.

[21] Parekh A K, Goodman RA, Gordon C, Koh HK, for The HHS Interagency Workgroup on Multiple Chronic Conditions. (2011): Managing multiple chronic conditions: a strategic framework for improving health outcomes and quality of life. Public Health Rep. 126:460-71.

[22] Smith SM, Soubhi H, Fortin M, Hudon C, O'Dowd T. (2012): Interventions for improving outcomes in patients with multimorbidity in primary care and community settings. Cochrane Database Syst Rev. 4:CD006560.

[23] Wallace E, Salisbury C, Guthrie B, Lewis C, Fahey T, Smith SM (2015): Managing patients with multimorbidity in primary care. BMJ 350:h176 doi: 10.1136/bmj.h176.

[24] Bodenheimer T, Wagner EH, Grunbach K. (2002): Improving primary care for patients with chronic illness. JAMA. 288:1775-79.

[25] Mills GD, Chambers CV. Effective strategies to improve the management of heart failure. Prim Care. 39(2):393-413.Epub 2012 Apr 24. Review.

[26] Kadu MK, Stolee P. (2015): Facilitators and barriers of implementing the chronic care model in primary care: a systematic review. BMC Fam Pract. 6;16:12.

[27] Murad K, Kitzman D. (2012): Frailty and multiple comorbidities in the elderly patient with heart failure: implications for management. Heart Fail Rev. 17(0): 581-588. doi: 10.1007/s10741-011-9258-y.

[28] Alagiakrishnan K, Banach M, Jones LG, Datta S, Ahmed A, Aronow WS. (2013): Update on diastolic heart failure or heart failure with preserved ejection fraction in the

older adults. Ann Med. 45(1):37-50. doi: 10.3109/07853890.2012.660493. Epub 2012 Mar 13.

[29] Allen LA, Stevenson LW, Grady KL, Goldstein NE, Matlock DD, Arnold RM et al. (2012): Decision making in advanced heart failure: a scientific statement from the American Heart Association. Circulation. 125:1928-52. doi:10.1161/CIR. 0b013e31824f2173.

[30] Kane PM, Murtagh FE, Ryan K, Mahon NG, McAdam B, McQuillan R, Ellis-Smith C, Tracey C, Howley C, Raleigh C, O'Gara G, Higginson IJ, Daveson BA. (2015): The gap between policy and practice: a systematic review of patient-centred care interventions in chronic heart failure. Heart Fail Rev. 20(6):673-87.

[31] Santurri LE. (2006): Patient Empowerment: Improving the Outcomes of Chronic Diseases Through Self Management Education. The MPHP 439 Online Text Book. Cleveland, Ohio: Case Western Reserve University.

[32] Battersby M, Von Korff M, Schaefer J, Davis C, Ludman E, Greene SM, Parkerton M, Wagner EH. (2010): Twelve evidence-based principles for implementing self-management support in primary care. Jt Comm J Qual Patient Saf. 36(12):561-70.

[33] Higgins R, Murphy B, Worcester M, Daffey A. (2012): Supporting chronic disease self-management: translating policies and principles into clinical practice. Aust J Prim Health. 18(1):80-7.

[34] Nolte S, Osborne RH. (2012): A systematic review of outcomes of chronic disease self-management interventions. Qual Life Res. 27. PMID: 23184454.

[35] Bartlett YK, Haywood A, Bentley CL, Parker J, Hawley MS, Mountain GA, Mawson S. (2014): The SMART personalised self-management system for congestive heart failure: results of a realist evaluation. BMC Med Inform Decis Mak. 14:109.

[36] Coulter A, Entwistle VA, Eccles A, Ryan S, Shepperd S, Perera R. (2015): Personalised care planning for adults with chronic or long-term health conditions. Cochrane Database Syst Rev. 3:CD010523.

[37] De Maria R, Misuraca G, Milli M, Filippi A. (2010): Role of outpatient heart failure clinics and primary care physicians in the tailored follow-up of heart failure patients. G Ital Cardiol (Rome). 11(5 Suppl 2):38S-44S. Italian.

[38] Cawley J, Grantham CC. Building a system of care: integration across the heart failure care continuum. Perm J. 15(3):37-42.

[39] Bentley A. Case management and long-term conditions: the evolution of community matrons. Br J Community Nurs. 19(7):340, 342-5. Review.

[40] Centeno MM, Kahveci KL. (2014): Transitional care models: preventing readmissions for high-risk patient populations. Crit Care Nurs Clin North Am. 26(4):589-97. Epub 2014 Sep 16.

[41] Dorling G, Fountaine T, McKenna S, Suresh B. (2015): The evidence for integrated care. Healthcare Practice.

[42] Murthy S, Lipman HI (2011): Management of end-stage heart failure. Prim Care. 38(2):265-76, viii. Review.

[43] Kul S, Barbieri A, Milan E, Montag I, Vanhaecht K, Panella M. (2012): Effects of care pathways on the in-hospital treatment of heart failure: a systematic review. BMC Cardiovasc Disord. 12:81. doi: 10.1186/1471-2261-12-81. Review.

[44] Erceg P, Despotovic N, Milosevic DP, Soldatovic I, Zdravkovic S, Tomic S, Markovic I, Mihajlovic G, Brajovic MD, Bojovic O, Potic B, Davidovic M. (2013): Health-related quality of life in elderly patients hospitalized with chronic heart failure. Clin Interv Aging. 8:1539-46. Epub 2013 Nov 15.

[45] Feitell S, Hankins SR, Eisen HJ. (2014): Adjunctive therapy and management of the transition of care in patients with heart failure. Cardiol Clin. 32(1):163-74, x. Review.

[46] Louis DZ, Robeson M, McAna J, Maio V, Keith SW, Liu M, Gonnella JS, Grilli R. (2014): Predicting risk of hospitalisation or death: a retrospective population-based analysis. BMJ Open. 4(9):e005223.

[47] Fendler TJ, Swetz KM, Allen LA. (2015): Team-based palliative and end-of-life care for heart failure. Heart Fail Clin. 11(3):479-98. Review.

[48] Jaarsma T, Larsen T, Strömberg A. (2013): Practical guide on home health in heart failure patients. Int J Integr Care. 13:e043. eCollection 2013.

[49] Martínez-González NA, Berchtold P, Ullman K, Busato A, Egger M. Integrated care programmes for adults with chronic conditions: a meta-review. Int J QualHealth Care. 26(5):561-70. Epub 2014 Aug 9. Review.

[50] Scottish Intercollegiate Guidelines Network (SIGN). Management of chronic heart failure. Edinburgh: SIGN; 2016. (SIGN publication no. 147). [March 2016]. Available from URL: http://www.sign.ac.uk.

Chapter 4

The Management of Dementia in Primary Care

Luc Pieter De Vreese, Luigi De Salvatore, Lara Rovesta and Andrea Fabbo

Additional information is available at the end of the chapter

http://dx.doi.org/10.5772/62762

Abstract

High-quality in-home primary healthcare services are pivotal for people with dementia and their families to avoid inappropriate hospital admissions and premature nursing home placement, which are associated with worsened quality of life of both the person with dementia and his family and financial burden.

This chapter gives a qualitative overview of the evidence on the efficacy and effectiveness of different primary care models covering all the stages of the disease from the onset of the disease until the more advanced stages with a particular focus on the management of behaviour and psychological disorders.

A detailed description is provided of the primary care model of the Province of Modena for people with dementia and their families in which the general practitioner plays a central role both in the diagnostic process and in follow-up and closely collaborates with first- and second-level healthcare professionals. This "collaborative care" network is able to address timely the continuously changing needs of these frail people and their caregivers, including acute severe behavioural and psychological disorders. A 10-item composite indicator of appropriateness of care by the general practitioner has been recently introduced to further improve the quality of care within primary care.

Keywords: Behavioural and psychological disorders, case-finding, models of primary care, dementia, family caregiver, cognitive screening tests

1. Introduction

Globally, the number of persons living with dementia (PWD) is projected to increase exponentially as population ages, becoming one of the most serious human, social, and economic

INTECH
open science | open minds

© 2016 The Author(s). Licensee InTech. This chapter is distributed under the terms of the Creative Commons Attribution License (http://creativecommons.org/licenses/by/3.0), which permits unrestricted use, distribution, and reproduction in any medium, provided the original work is properly cited.

burdens of this century. According to the World Alzheimer Report 2015 [1] it is estimated that 46.8 million people around the world live with dementia now and that this number will almost double every 20 years. At present, the estimated global incidence of dementia is 9.9 million new cases, implying one new case every 3.2 seconds. The most recent population based prevalence study in Italy [2] shows that one quarter of 80+ year old people have dementia, most of them in the advanced stages of the disease with prevalence rates that continue to rise gradually even in extreme ages: 15.7% in people aged 80–84 years to 52.8% and 65.9% in people aged 95–99 and in centenarians, respectively [2]. Also the incidence rates of dementia per 100 person-years do not level off but increase gradually ranging from 6 person-years at 80–84 years to 20–21 person-years at 95–99 years (Lucca U et al., unpublished data).

Dementia is defined as a progressive major neurocognitive syndromal (group of signs/ symptoms) disorder characterised by neuropsychological impairments, reduced ability to perform activities in everyday life and behavioural and psychological symptoms of dementia (BPSD). These deficits cause significant impairment in social or occupational functioning and represent a significant decline from a previous level of functioning [3].

The progression of the disease greatly differs from one type to another, but most types of dementia are characterised by an early loss of declarative memory and progressive deficits in other cognitive domains (*e.g.*, executive function, language, abstract reasoning) significantly interfering with overall daily-live functioning. In addition, over 90% of PWD manifest at least one challenging behaviour or clinically relevant psychological symptom during the course of their disease [4].

The increasing number of PWD will lead to a rising demand for informal and formal care services in order to attend to the needs of this group of people. The possibility of getting support depends on numerous interrelated factors such as patients' and carers' (socio-economic) characteristics, care setting, provision of services, availability of healthcare providers and the degree of integration among care networks. Some research suggests that co-habitant family caregivers (CGs) could be replacing formal support services provided that they accept supervision or advice from social and primary healthcare services. Unfortunately, many CGs do not connect their relative with social and healthcare professionals, which may constitute a disadvantage for both of them [5]. There are different reasons why CGs do not search formal support among which the principal are stigma surrounding dementia, CGs' perceived lack of need and support, PWD's refusal to accept help, service characteristics and lack of knowledge about service availability [6, 7]. All these findings show PWD as a vulnerable group. Developing interventions, such as case/care management which allow the coordination between different agents involved in community care might offer the possibility necessary to satisfy the needs of PWD and their CGs in the primary care context [8].

Obstacles to detecting dementia at the primary care level include limited time resources [9–13], insufficient expertise, flaw in skill set, fear of making an erroneous diagnosis, unsatisfactory reimbursement, and deficiencies in the coordination between family physicians (henceforth called general practitioners (GPs)) and community services [14–18].

Not surprisingly, two-thirds of all dementia and 91% of incipient dementia remain undetected in the primary care setting around the world. Even when GPs accurately recognise dementia, the quality of management of the disease after the diagnosis frequently appears suboptimal. Initiation of dementia-specific drug treatment [19], assessment and management of BPSD, safety issues, side effects of psychotropic drugs and of CGs' stress and burden [20], coordination of primary healthcare partners [21], implementation of support for PWD and their CGs [22] represent the main challenges for providing quality dementia care by the GPs. Inadequacies in the diagnosis and management of dementia have been found to increase the risk for hospitalisation and nursing home placement contributing substantially to the economic burden of dementia [23].

Different models of care have been designed to help GPs in detecting dementia and in delivering better dementia care. Research in this field has yielded to date mixed results in terms of efficiency and effectiveness [24–28]. In contrast, a collaborative care model in which an interdisciplinary team works with both the PWD and the CG, and which is integrated with a primary care network, improves adherence to dementia care guidelines and reduces BPSD of the PWD and stress and depression of their CGs [29, 30]. Although limited in scope, research suggests that including geriatric specialists in the detection of dementia increases the rates of screening people for dementia [18]. In a recent exploratory study [31], dementia care was delivered through a system involving three groups of healthcare providers: (a) GPs involved in the primary care network for identification and management of dementia; (b) a geriatric assessment team (a GP who had extensive training in geriatrics and nurses specialised in assessing frail elderly) and (c) community care composed of nurses and other healthcare professionals (e.g., social workers, occupational therapists, psychologists). The geriatric assessment team assisted with the evaluation of the PWD and with client-tailored care planning (exhaustive listing of problems, recommendations, multidomain interventions and follow-up). Community care delivered personal support services to the PWD and their families integrated with the primary care network. Although it was assumed that this current approach to caring for PWD would have resulted in high-quality dementia care, a retrospective analysis of the charts of these three groups of healthcare providers evidenced several gaps and inconsistencies, underscoring the need of further research to assess whether the overall quality of dementia diagnosis and management at the primary care level may be achieved through a collaborative model that integrates different healthcare services [31–33].

2. Early diagnosis and case finding in primary care; the diagnostic burden.

Despite the worldwide increased recognition of the early symptoms of dementia, this disease still remains too often a hidden problem, especially in resource-limited communities. Many family members do not seek help, and GPs seldom come across cases (see below) because loss of memory and other related cognitive functions are thought to be part of an usual cognitive aging process (i.e., ageism) and not a medical (i.e., pathological) condition. Dementia, however, is a significant source of burden both for the PWD and his/her family. Hence, more research on interventions to promote help-seeking behaviour and to improve the diagnostic expertise of non-specialist healthcare providers, is urgently needed. For instance, it is mandatory to compare the accuracy of the clinical evaluations done by these first- and second-level healthcare providers against a standard assessment process for the diagnosis of dementia by a specialist. If it could be shown that a network of non-specialist healthcare providers is able to reliably identify dementia cases in the community and in the primary care setting, then it might deliver simple and effective interventions in these settings with supervision and counselling as needed by the specialists [34].

GPs are usually the first health professionals that either patients or their families contact if concerned about memory decline. However only 60% of the people who meet the diagnostic criteria receive a formal diagnosis of dementia: failure rates have been estimated between 50% and 80% for moderate-to-severe dementia and up to 91% for mild cases. Yet, owing to their long relationship with patients (and their families), GPs are in a favourable and unique position to collect the information needed to define the patient's cognitive, functional and behavioural profile. This is pivotal not only for the diagnostic process but also for care planning tailored to the needs of the PWD and his/her family and for the assessment of treatment effects. GPs underdiagnose dementia for several reasons; apart from those already mentioned above, there is also the limited availability of guidelines specific for the GP's practice that might allow to better approach the diagnostic burden of dementia, especially in its early stages [34, 35].

Although general practice is usually the first point of contact for patients with memory problems or other symptoms of dementia, GPs appear reluctant to use brief cognitive tests and to refer patients for early assessment, particularly in disadvantaged older people with functional impairment [36]. On the other hand, there is increasing evidence that people want earlier diagnosis, with younger healthcare professionals perceiving its usefulness and the international guidelines emphasising the importance of early diagnosis [37–40]. In primary care there is a need to develop training in assessment so that clinicians are more aware of dementia to deliver a timely diagnosis [41]. Studies based on a focus-group methodology about practitioners' knowledge have shown that primary care recognition can be enhanced; however, this does not always result in greater adherence to practice guidelines [42]. Education should also include assessment of GPs' needs, otherwise facilitation of system change does not improve performance or health outcomes and it is suggested that small group education is important. A 'whole system' approach has been advocated to improve self-management of long-term conditions, but interventions have limited impact on patients' outcomes [43, 44].

Across the European Union more than 50% of PWD never receive a specialist diagnosis or do so only at the late stage of disease or at a time of crisis, despite an growing evidence that early diagnosis and subsequent interdisciplinary intervention are cost-effective [45, 46]. Early diagnosis in dementia within primary care is important as this allows PWD, their CGs and care networks to set up support services and to act proactively for the future, in accordance with the adage of "spend to save". The North of England Evidence Based Dementia Guideline Development Group states that *'population screening for dementia in the over 65s is not recommended; a case finding approach is recommended'*. It makes the recommendation that GPs should consider using formal cognitive testing to enhance their clinical judgment [47]. However, the development group fails to recommend which tests to use and how often to use them throughout the elderly population at risk. Although this group, despite its name, makes recommendations based on the clinical opinions of GPs, recommendations based on evidence are given more weight by some US organizations [48].

A number of *simple tools are available* for use in the community to make an initial assessment of a patient's cognitive function [49]. The most commonly used cognitive assessment tool is the *Mini-Mental State Examination* (MMSE); marked out of 30, a score of less than 25 is suggestive of dementia [50]. However, this examination can take up to 15–20 minutes to complete and may not be practical for use within a primary care consultation, which is usually allocated just 10 minutes. The *General Practitioner Assessment of Cognition* (GPCOG) [51] and two other cognitive screening tests, the *Mini-Cog Assessment Instrument* [52] and the *Memory Impairment Screen* (MIS) [53], have been found to be as clinically and psychometrically robust and more appropriate for use in primary care than the MMSE. The GPCOG is estimated to take 5 to 7 minutes to complete, with questions for both the patient and carer to answer, making it more relevant for GPs. An alternative, developed in primary care, is the *Six-Item Cognitive Impairment Test* (6-CIT), which performs as well as the MMSE, but is easier to use [54]. The administration of a *clock-drawing test* (CDT) may also be a useful quick and simple test for the GP's routine practice [55]. A short video produced by the *American College of Physicians Foundation* and the *Alzheimer's Association* demonstrates how to use the Mini-Cog for the assessment of cognitive impairment during a primary care visit [56]. In addition, an 8-item informant tool called the *AD8* is a very useful method of gathering information from someone who knows the patient well [57]. A recent systematic review suggests that if length is not a major consideration, the MMSE [50] may remain the best tool for primary care clinicians who want to make a syndromal diagnosis of dementia [58].

Yet, another recent evidence-based recommendation on *Practical Diagnosis and Management of Dementia due to Alzheimer's disease in the primary care setting* does not advocate the MMSE as a screening test because of its length, education and literacy biases, and financial burden due to copyright issues [59]. As no single cognitive screening tool can actually be considered the gold standard, a reasonable proposal may be to familiarise with one of the above listed suitable instruments and incorporate it into routine practice [60].

Technology platforms such as diagnostic support aids, offer an important solution but need further research as there are accuracy and reliability issues with subsequent reduced help-seeking behaviours due to false–negative results, or generating unnecessary distress with false-positive results [61]. A recent proposal from the *Italian Society of General Practitioners* (SIMG) to improve early diagnosis of dementia in general practice, reviewed the literature and ascertained the contributing factors for GPs' missed or delayed diagnosis of dementia (Table 1), the **Brief Psychometric Screening Tools** with an administration time <5 minutes and with negative predictive values superior to those of the MMSE (Table 2) and the guidelines targeted for GPs' detection of dementia [62–69].

The identification of possible cases of dementia in the primary healthcare setting and in the community needs medical practice-based educational programmes and awareness-raising campaigns. Short informant questionnaires and cognitive tests should be used to confirm these cases. A formal diagnosis of a probable primary progressive dementia at first- or second-healthcare level can be made only after an exhaustive past and present medical review, included drug therapy and alcohol abuse in order to rule out other common (reversible) causes of cognitive impairment and decline [60–69].

Cultural barriers	1. Absent/limited education during undergraduate or postgraduate training in Medicine 2. Ageism: GPs who attribute cognitive complaints to age; patients or families lacking insight and not referring for assessment
Clinical variability	Dementia subtypes develop slowly, in years. Many of their early clinical pictures may be insidious due to slight differences with normal ageing. Failure to recognise BPSD, if these are the first signs before obvious memory complaints/disorders or functional impairment.
Practical issues	Lack of time, financial resources and GP-focussed guidelines

Reproduced with permission from Pirani et al., 2011 [69].

Table 1. The diagnostic burden of dementia for GPs

Test	Orientation	Memory		Praxis, visuospatial	Aphasia, verbal fluency	Functional status from informant	Cross-cultural validation
		STM & LTM	General information				
AMT	X	X	X				
CDT				X			X
CP-COG	X	X		X	X	X	X
SPSMQ	X		X				X
6-CIT	X	X					
Mini-COG		X		X			
MIT		X					
BAS	X	X			X		

Adapted with permission from Pirani et al., 2011 [69].

AMT, Abbreviated Mental Test; CDT, Clock Drawing Test; CP-COG, General Practitioner Assessment of Cognition; SPMSQ, Short Portable Mental State Questionnaire; 6-CIT, 6-Item Cognitive Impairment Test; Mini-COG, Mini Cognitive Assessment Instrument; MIS, Memory Impairment Screen and BAS, Brief Alzheimer Screen.

Table 2. Selection of brief psychometric screening tests.

3. The collaborative model for dementia in primary care

As outlined above, collaborative care for the treatment of dementia resulted in a significant improvement in the quality of care and in BPSD among primary care patients and their CGs. These improvements were achieved without significantly increasing the use of antipsychotics or sedative-hypnotics [29]. Indeed, BPSD represent a major challenge in the care of PWD. These symptoms, which include a broad range of distressing behaviours and psychological reactions, affect the health and quality of life of both the PWD and his/her CG. BPSD are not simply a manifestation of advanced dementia. For instance, behavioural abnormalities are reported in 35–75% of people with mild cognitive impairment with the most common being depression, apathy, anxiety and irritability [70]. Leaving patients' BPSD untreated, undertreated or treated improperly has been associated with patients' excess disability, poor management of comorbid conditions, increased hospitalisation rates, premature institutionalisation, suffering for both the PWD and the CG and substantial increase in financial costs.

Some studies compared the effectiveness of collaborative care management with usual care for older PWD with comorbidity or multimorbidity that is typically found in primary care. The extreme heterogeneity of the targeted population and the fact that this model starts from the perspective of the GP probably explain a major treatment effect on BPSD rather than on the other domains of dementia like cognition and everyday functioning [71, 72].

In the context of collaborative dementia care models (or others models of in-home care services such as *integrated care*, *consumer directed care* and *restorative care*) [73] psychosocial interventions play a leading role. Psychosocial interventions in dementia are nonpharmacological approaches involving interactions between people to support cognition, emotion, meaningful activity and interpersonal relationships. They aim to enhance or maintain quality of life by maximising psychological and social function in the context of existing disabilities [74]. Effective psychosocial interventions are usually multicomponent, individualised and targeted to the context and personal needs of both the PWD and his/her family [74, 75]. A range of individually tailored approaches have been developed including cognitive stimulation, cognitive rehabilitation, reminiscence therapy, emotion-based care [76] and adaptations from standard psychological therapies such as cognitive behaviour therapy which can be used with the person and/or the carer to reframe experiences of dementia and thus improve quality of life and coping with the condition [77, 78]. Other approaches include involving pets, music, dance, exercise and art therapies, although the evidence for these has yet to be established. Group-based support in community dementia care albeit an intuitively popular approach is so far only weakly evidence-based. An exception is cognitive stimulation therapy, an activity and discussion group therapy that aims to improve quality of life by enhancing cognitive and social functioning [79–81] and it has been recommended 'for all people with mild to moderate dementia' by the NICE Guidelines for Dementia, although not all PWD want to engage in group therapy. Psychosocial interventions that help PWD and families to cope with changing roles and relationships and that teach ways to minimise the impact of dementia are an important focus for those in dementia care [82]. Individualised interventions such as *cognitive rehabilitation* [83] and *occupational therapy* [84] usually involving family or friends helping the PWD to achieve their goals in life, *remain an important avenue for the future of psychosocial interventions in dementia primary care*. Such interventions can also have components to meet the needs of the family carers [85]. The implementation of psychosocial interventions in primary care often focus on educational interventions for GPs, although studies of the quality of care in primary care suggest that more psychosocial approaches can be undertaken [86] with the application of carefully developed quality indicators for the delivery of dementia care [87].

The paucity of research in psychosocial approaches in primary care presumably stems from a poor understanding of the value of psychosocial interventions in community settings [88]. Information provision is seen as a key to dementia care support but this does not appear to be done timely or tailored to the constantly changing needs of PWD and their families. This may be because of the application of a medical management model where a social disability framework for delivering support in primary care is more relevant in guiding dementia care practice [89]. For these reasons the management of PWD and their CGs should be organised on the *model of integrated care*, described as "*the management and delivery of health services so that clients receive a continuum of preventive and curative services, according to their needs over time and across different levels of the health system*" [90].

In primary care, the *medication management* is a key element of providing optimal care for PWD [91]. The current focus has been on the use of first- and second-generation antipsychotics to treat challenging behaviours and the recent UK guidelines targeted a reduction in such usage by two-thirds [92]. However, effective medication management in dementia is much broader than just the appropriate treatment of BPSD. PWD may rely upon informal carers to manage their medication and these carers may conduct various medication management activities, including the recognition and management of side effects and the decision to administer or not medication [93]. GPs should be aware that dementia increases the likelihood that key risk factors—including inappropriate prescribing, old age, adherence issues, drug interactions, comorbidity or multimorbidity and polypharmacy—for medication-related adverse events are present [94]. Medication errors may be more common in PWD because of the involvement of multiple health and social care professionals; the primary–secondary care interface may be particularly risky [95]. Specific factors including frailty and comorbidity or multimorbidity may increase the risk of adverse reactions. Falls are a major cause of injury in older people [96]. Psychotropic drugs including antidepressants, neuroleptics and benzodiazepines belong to one of the main groups of medications associated with falls, the so-called 'fall risk increased drugs' (FRID). Polypharmacy is also a risk factor for falls and older people should have regular medication reviews. If possible, psychotropics and other unnecessary medicines should be discontinued to reduce the risk of a fall. There is also increasing evidence that treatments specifically administered for the symptoms of dementia cause falls. Cholinesterase inhibitors (ChEI) notably cause bradycardia, arterial hypotension or hypertension, syncope and dizziness with increased fall risk and hip fracture [97]. If family carers are not aware of the potential link, they may continue to administer ChEI despite a recent history of falling in the patient. In summary, safe and effective medication management in dementia is complex and difficult to achieve. A collaborative approach that improves outcomes by linking primary and secondary healthcare services—including general practice and pharmacy—with social care needs to be developed. A key outcome of such a collaborative approach would be to support informal CGs to optimise the management of medication.

4. The case management model in primary care

PWD and their CGs often encounter services that are fragmented, protocol-driven and only weakly tailored to individual and family needs. Because dementia is a more or less slowly progressive disease, the needs of the PWD may change greatly over time, requiring consequently support from a complex and flexible matrix of social networks and services, as well as from family CGs who should adapt themselves to the cumulative repercussions inherent to the disease (and associated chronic or new onset) organic pathologies of their relative with dementia. In addition, the interaction of medical professionals, PWD, family, and systems barriers in primary and secondary care explain why providing timely, proactive, responsive, well-coordinated and patient-centred clinical care is so difficult [9, 98].

In Europe, there is a great need to reconfigure services for PWD and their families so that they become more patient-centred and family-centred. Case management approaches that start with an assessment of needs shared between patients, caregivers and professionals, show promise as a way to improve the quality of life of PWD and their families, reduce health expenditure (e.g., inappropriate hospital admissions), and produce societal gains [99]. A recent systematic review of randomised controlled trials (RCTs) of case management for PWD and their CGs concluded that the evidence for the efficacy of case management with reference to cost and resource usage is not strong enough and that further studies ought to consider who might benefit more from case management [98]. On the other hand, some well-conducted, long-term studies have demonstrated how case management can delay institutionalisation, with potentially important health and economic gains [100–103].

Case management was found to not affect nursing home placement, hospitalisation and emergency room (ER) referrals [104], and consistent with this, the reviews agreed that case management produced small to no decreases in resource utilisation when healthcare expenditure, hospitalisation or institutionalisation were considered [105]. There is a limited number of RCTs of in-home care/case management for PWD. These studies measured a diversity of outcomes that makes it difficult to draw conclusions. A Finnish study found that case management was effective in deferring nursing home placement, particularly for persons with severe dementia; however, by the end of the 2-years follow-up, the numbers of participants admitted to long-term residential care were similar for case management and usual care groups [106]. An American study over 12 months found that in comparison with usual care, case-managed clients improved adherence and quality of care on dementia guidelines, increased use of community agency assistance, and patient health–related quality of life, overall quality of patient care, caregiving quality, social support and level of unmet caregiving assistance needs [101].

Another study found that characteristics of case management, which negatively influence implementation, are low intensity of case management (e.g., infrequent follow-up), a large case load (60 patients or more per case manager), and a reactive (rather than proactive) approach to care [107]. In the Netherlands, the model of case management in which case manager and client services are embedded *within one type of organisation* is more successful in facilitating implementation of care compared to the model where the case manager coordinates services from a range of organisations. In summary, case management for PWD may increase the use of community-based services and delay nursing home admission [74].

There is a great need to reconfigure services for PWD and their families to become more patient- centred, using case management approaches that start with an assessment of needs shared between PWD, CGs and healthcare professionals. The Case Management Society of the United Kingdom defines case management as *"a collaborative process which assesses, plans, implements, co-ordinates, monitors and evaluates the options and services required to meet an individual's health, and social care, educational and employment needs, using communication and available resources to promote quality cost effective outcomes"*[98]. Case management, as a clinical management technique, offers a way of creating patient-centred interventions and has been shown to be effective for some people with multiple or single long-term care needs. However, the diffusion of case management methods has been very variable, and there is a need to overcome the block that impedes the transfer of knowledge into practice.

5. The "Modena Primary Care Dementia Project"

5.1. Historical overview

In 1999 the Regional Government of Emilia-Romagna deliberated the "Regional Dementia Project" (D.G.R. 2581/1999), an act that provides funds for the organisation of Health and Social Welfare Services in the community for PWD aimed at (a) ensuring a correct and timely diagnosis of dementia; (b) ameliorating the health-related quality of life and overall quality of care of PWD; (c) extending the period of home care for as long as possible; (d) adapting, expanding and specialising the existing health and social network services for PWD; (e) enhancing the role of the family associations and (f) qualifying the care processes of hospitalised PWD. The regional project's actions to guarantee global care plans, follow-up and continuity of (in-home) care of PWD include (a) creation of a network of specialist centres for cognitive disorders and dementia (CCDD) with competencies in diagnosis and care planning; (b) increase of formal and informal support for families of PWD; (c) amelioration of the network services tailored to the individual needs and resources of the individual PWD and his/her CGs and (d) widespread training and education of social and healthcare professionals.

According to this regional dementia project, and given the GP's pivotal role in the timely diagnosis of dementia, the Local Authority for Health (*Azienda Sanitaria Locale*, ASL) of Modena and the Department of Primary Care together with the most representative GPs' organisations, implemented in 2002 a targeted protocol, called "Cognitive Disorders Project," to involve on voluntary basis GPs in dementia screening by means of accreditation courses promoting an uniform screening assessment. In 2007, the Director of the Health Thrust of the ASL of Modena approved a new agreement with the GPs consisting of a protocol for taking care of PWD and their families by the GP and the CCDDs. This renewed protocol is aimed at improving (a) integrated care of PWD through a more fruitful and assiduous dialogue between the GP and CCDDs already from the start of the diagnostic process of dementia (b) follow-up with ongoing monitoring of the treatment schedules for ChEI, Memantine and second-generation antipsychotics (olanzapine, risperidone, quetiapine, clozapine) according to note 85 of the *Agenzia Italiana del Farmaco* (AIFA, Italian Agency of Drugs) and of the overall healthcare of PWD (c) the effective role of the GPs as consultants, with particular reference to BPSD in crisis situations and (d) health and non-health in-home care of PWD in the more advanced stages of the disease avoiding unnecessary ER referrals, hospitalisation and premature nursing home placement.

The final outcome of these two protocols are to improve the quality of life and health of PWD and their families, satisfying the preference of PWD (and/or their families) to remain living at home and maintain normality for as long as possible deferring long-term residential care in agreement with the results of some RCTs of integrated care models for the frail elderly including people with cognitive impairment [108].

5.2. Dementia case-finding (Form A)

When the GP suspects an incipient dementia, he/she administers the *Symptom of Dementia Screener* (SDS) [109] and the MMSE [50]. When the SDS score is ≥5 and the MMSE score is <26, GP quantifies the patient's somatic comorbidity by means of the *Cumulative Illness Rating Scale* (CIRS) [110] and his functional efficiency through the administration of the IADL [111] and ADL [112] scales. In addition, the GP prescribes blood chemistries and instrumental examination, as suggested by the international diagnostic guidelines such as the DSM-IV-TR [113]. Once collected all the above information, including anamnesis regarding family history of dementia, past or present psychiatric diseases or alcohol abuse and current drug therapy, the GP refers the patient with the completed Form A in all its parts to one of the 10 specialist CCDDs present in the Province of Modena for a differential diagnosis (usual cognitive aging, different types of mild cognitive impairment, dementia with a typological diagnosis), therapy and care planning. As needed, the family may be referred to a clinical psychologist for individual or group counselling.

5.3. Follow up (Form B)

After the diagnostic work-up, the patient is returned to the care of the referring GP with (typological) diagnosis and advices for follow-up with annual compilation of Form B which includes, in addition to the patient's cognitive (MMSE), functional ([I]ADL) and physical health (CIRS) status, data regarding the recourse to day centre or (temporary respite) residential care and the implementation of a " health in-home care service" integrated with local public or private social service systems (the so-called *Assistenza Domiciliare Integrata,* ADI). The GP also reports the presence of psychological distress of the family CGs and may plan psychological and/or social support according to the following eligibility criteria: the context or consequences of caregiving and of well-being and treatment motivation of the family carer.

The following paragraphs illustrate some results of the most relevant aspects of the Modena Project collected in 2013.

5.4. GPs' adhesion to the project

About 68% (385 out of 568) of the GPs practicing in the 7 Health Districts of the Province of Modena are actively participating into this project on completely voluntary but remunerated basis. Between 2007 and 2013, 9542 PWD have been enrolled by the GPs (Form A and B) with 5195 cases (females = 64.5%; median age = 86 years) still active (Form B for follow-up) in 2013.

5.5. GPs' referral for diagnosis to the specialist centres

Of 4530 outpatients referred by the GPs for the first time to the specialist of CCDDs, 2778 patients received a diagnosis of dementia (61%), whereas 865 patients (20%) were considered at risk (mild cognitive/vascular impairment). Only 598 cases (14%) did not display any sign/ symptom of cognitive impairment or dementia. Though these figures suggest an appropriate referral by GPs to the specialist of CCDD, it should be noted that in reality only 8% of PWD aged 65–80 years and 48% of PWD with age >80 years are enrolled by the GPs according to the estimated prevalence of dementia in these two age subgroups (i.e., 4% and 16.8% respectively) (data from the Department of Clinical Epidemiology of Modena, unpublished), confirming the universally observed trend to underdiagnose dementia in primary care.

5.6. Ordinary and semi-urgent home visits

In 2013, 3706 home visits (i.e., at home, in nursing homes and in day care centres) have been conducted, some of them together with GPs, which correspond to 22% of the total (first and control) visits (n= 16,623), confirming the important work done by the CCDDs at the provincial level as part of the Department of Primary Care. As presented in Table 3, eligibility criteria for ordinary and semi-urgent home visits have been established in agreement between the specialists of the CCDDs and the GPs. An analysis of the 65 "semi-urgent" home visit requests received by the CCDD of the Health District of Modena in the first half of 2014 is as follows. Only 8 of 65 requests were followed by a home visit within 7 working days from the GPs' phone call; 9 requests were resolved with a telephone conversation between the referring GP and the Geriatrician; 26 cases have been turned into "semi-urgent outpatient visits" at the CCDD and 22 in ordinary home visits. In 12 PWD (18.5%), it was necessary to activate other services: one patient was sent to the ER, one to a territorial Centre of Mental Health, three patients were assessed by a Multidimensional Assessment Unit—a team composed of a Geriatrician, a Nurse and a Social Worker—two patients were transferred to a Special Hospital Unit (SHU) for Dementia, three to an Alzheimer Day Centre (ADC) and two to a temporary residential Special Care Unit (SCU). The latter three structures are an integral part of the integrated network of health and social services dedicated to the diagnosis and treatment of PWD with BPSD related to dementia, environment or caregiving (ADC and SCU) or secondary to organic or iatrogenic comorbidities or multimorbidities (SHU) according to the evidenced-based model of structures and organisations for the care of major BPSD (Alzheimer Cooperative Valuation in Europe, www.alcove-project.eu).

5.7. Integrated domiciliary care

As explained above, the Modena project pays great attention to support PWD in their own homes. In-home care for PWD is delivered in close cooperation with the treating GP across the province through a wide range of actions (see Figure 1) ranging from the aforementioned agreement act with the GPs for taking care of PWD and their families to the use of respite care (nursing homes, SCU, ADC) and to an economic support (care voucher)—similar to the consumer-directed care model— thanks to regional funds for long-term care of frail elderly for low-income families who decide to care for their loved at home.

Health and social services intervene whenever one of the following trigger conditions is verified (a) the PWD lives alone without direct relatives and a valid homemaker assistance; (b) home environment requires adaptation to the PWD's new onset needs; (c) family or formal CGs are in trouble and unable to manage BPSD; (d) the PWD's clinical picture or social conditions undergo a substantial worsening that requires the search for an alternative care plan and (e) the PWD evolves to a terminal stage of illness.

· Bedridden patient or with major locomotion difficulties (rendering a problematic transport to the CCDD) · Patient with preserved ambulation but frankly uncooperative and/or depressed who refuses to leave the house	
Ordinary home visits	Semi-urgent home visits (within 7 working days)
Persistent BPSD: aberrant motor activity, vocalizations, physical aggression, insomnia	Persistent (for at least 10 days), major and worsening BPSD: aberrant motor activity, continuous vocalizations, physical aggression, delusions and/or hallucinations with functional impact, insomnia)
Exclusion criteria: · Organic precipitating causes such as infection or uncontrolled pain (e.g., (S)DSD) · BPSD refractory to drug therapy and psychosocial interventions already undertaken before	

CCDD, centre for cognitive disorders and dementia; BPSD, behavioural and psychological symptoms of dementia and (S)DSD, (subsyndromal) *delirium* superimposed on dementia.

Table 3. Inclusion and exclusion criteria for ordinary and semi-urgent home visits

The latter service is delivered provided that the following conditions are met (a) inability to easily reach points of care; (b) the presence of at least a prevalent organic symptom (e.g., aspiration pneumonia); (c) presumed life expectations inferior to 4 months; (d) little opportunity to intervene with effective care and (e) family CGs are adequate and are integrated with the healthcare team.

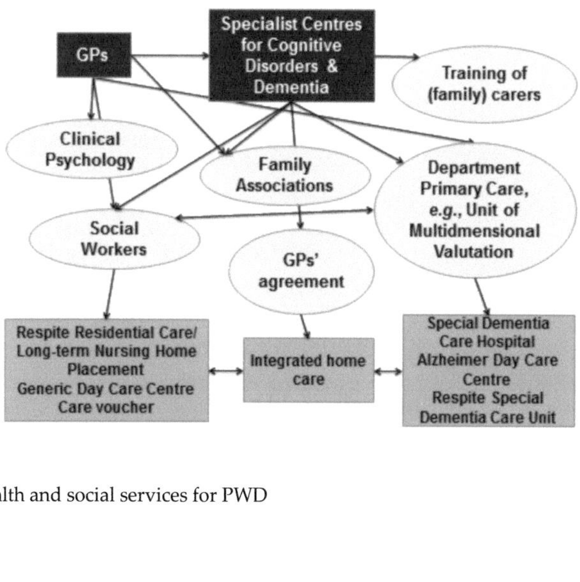

Figure 1. Network of health and social services for PWD

In 2013, 2210 PWD have been followed in domiciliary care, representing 42% of the total number of PWD (5,195 forms B still active) cared for in the long term by the GPs. This percentage highlights how the use of in-home care is becoming an increasingly necessary care model for PWD, especially in the end-stage of the disease. Indeed, an analysis of the nursing care activities documents a prevalence of interventions for complications typical of late-stage dementia, such as the treatment of pressure ulcers (representing 44% of total domiciliary nurse activities). Overall these data indicate that dementia has become the second most important disease (after chronic heart failure, but before cancer disease) in contrast to what happened before where cancer care at home exceeded that for dementia.

5.8. The Modena project: from the present to the future

The next step of the Modena project is the introduction of an indicator of the quality of care of PWD in primary care as suggested also by the recent National Dementia Plan (October 2014). The intention is to substitute the hard-copy reports (Form B) with manual extraction of data with an electronic format provided by a software house containing, besides information about demographic and clinical data, additional biochemical and instrumental tests and pharmaceutical treatment (Table 4).

		0 points	5 points	10 points	Source
1	Presence of PEG/feeding tube	YES	--	NO	ADI web/CCI/ABC software for NH
2	Use of antipsychotics	YES > 90 days of therapy/year	YES but > 90 days of therapy/year	NO	ADI web/CCI/ABC software for NH
3	HbA1c in diabetes mellitus	HbA1c < 6,5% o > 8,5%	6,5%<HbA1c < 7,5%	7,5 % < HbA1c < 8,5% or No Diabetes mellitus	CCI
4	Use of benzodiazepines or hypnotics	Yes > 30 days of therapy/year	Yes but ≤30 days of therapy/year	No	CCI
5	Use of fluoroquinolones	YES	YES but ≤ 2 blisters/ year	No	CCI
6	1 ECG/year in patients who uses antipsychotics	No	--	Yes or No antipsychotic therapy	CCI
7	1 creatinemia /year	No	--	Yes	CCI
8	Blood Pressure (BP) Measurement	No	BP< 110/70 mmHg BP> 140/90 mmHg	110/70 mmHg<BP< 140/90 mmHg	CCI
9	1 NPI/year	No	--	Yes	CCI/CCDD
10	1 PAINAD/year	No	--	Yes	CCI/CCDD

CCI, medical records data; CCDD, centre for cognitive disorders and dementia; ADI, health in-home care; NH nursing home; NPI, neuropsychiatric inventory and PAINAD, pain in advanced dementia.

Table 4. The QUADISC composite indicator

http://dx.doi.org/10.5772/62762

The collected data will be integrated and assembled into a single database and analysed in collaboration with the Department of Clinical Epidemiology of the ASL of Modena, in order to develop a reporting, including the introduction of a composite indicator of quality of care, following the recommendations of the "*Choosing Wisely*" of the American Geriatrics Society [114, 115] and from other evidence-based medicine data in elderly PWD [116–123].

This composite indicator, called QuADisC (*Qualità dell'Assistenza al paziente con Disturbi Cognitivi,* Quality of care of the patient with cognitive disorders), consists of 10 items (Table 4). For each item a score of 0, 5 or 10 is assigned, respectively, for non-target (or missing data), partially or fully achieved action on the part of the GP. The sum produces an overall score (maximum 100) that is directly proportional to the effectiveness of the care of the PWD.

For each patient, the total score will be calculated automatically within a clinical database that integrates demographic information and other clinical data provided by the GPs. There will be a refunding for the GP who sends the required data.

The QuADisC will be validated by correlating with an indicator of the effectiveness of care based on the number of (a) ER visits, (b) hospital admissions; (c) nursing home placement and (d) mortality, specifying reasons of ER referrals, admission to acute hospital wards or a nursing home and possibly the cause of the *exitus*.

6. Conclusions

Primary care is pivotal to the delivery of good quality assessment and care for PWD. There is a need for greater dementia-specific awareness through education and the organisation of systems both within practices and across interfaces between organisations. There are at least three specific areas that need addressing to improve care of PWD in primary care (1) necessity to standardise assessment tools and to use innovative technologies to facilitate early diagnosis; (2) opportunity to increase awareness of the benefits of psychosocial interventions in primary care for PWD, such as psychological interventions for CGs, cognitive stimulation and occupational therapy and (3) possibility to promote knowledge on the use of drugs by PWD and an enhancement of supportive strategies for patients and carers.

It is hoped that the introduction of a "*collaborative model,*" such as the 'Modena network' (Figure 1), with measurable indicators of appropriateness of care by the GP (see QuADisC, Table 4) will further improve the quality of care for PWD and their CGs in the context of primary care.

Author details

Luc Pieter De Vreese*, Luigi De Salvatore, Lara Rovesta and Andrea Fabbo*

*Address all correspondence to: l.devreese@ausl.mo.it; a.fabbo@ausl.mo.it

Dementia Programme, Health Trust, Local Authority for Health of Modena (ASL), Modena, Italy

References

[1] Alzheimer's Disease International. *The Global Impact of Dementia. An analysis of prevalence, incidence, cost and trends.* London: Alzheimer's Disease International (ADI), 2015.

[2] Lucca U, Tettamanti M, Tiraboschi P, et al. Prevalence of dementia in the oldest old: the Monzino 80-plus population based study. *Alzheimers Dement* 2015;11:258–70.

[3] American Psychiatric Association. *Diagnostic and statistical manual of mental disorders.* (5th ed.). Washington, DC: American Psychiatric Association, 2013.

[4] Steinberg M, Shao H, Zandi P, et al. Point and 5-year period prevalence of neuropsychiatric symptoms in dementia: the Cache County Study. *Int J Geriatr Psychiatry* 2008;23:170–7.

[5] Nelson T, Livingston G, Knapp M, Manela M, Kitchen G, Katona C. Slicing the health service cake: the Islington study. *Age Ageing* 2002;31:445–50.

[6] Moriarty JM. Use of community and long-term care by people with dementia in the UK: a review of some issues in service provision and carer and user preferences. *Aging Ment Health* 1999;3:311–9.

[7] Brodaty H, Thomson C, Thompson C, Fine M. Why caregivers of people with dementia and memory loss don't use services. *Int J Geriatr Psychiatry* 2005;20:537–46.

[8] Reilly S, Miranda-Castillo C, Sandhu S, Hoe J, Challis D, Orrell M. Case management approaches to home support for people with dementia. *Cochrane Database Syst Rev* 2015;1:CD008345.

[9] Koch T, Iliffe S. Rapid appraisal of barriers to the diagnosis and management of patients with dementia in primary care: a systematic review. *BMC Fam Pract* 2010;11:52.

[10] Van Hout H, Vernooij-Dassen M, Bakker K, Blom M, Grol R. General practitioners on dementia: tasks, practices and obstacles. *Patient Educ Couns* 2000;39:219–25.

[11] Bradford A, Kunik ME, Schulz P, Williams SP, Singh H. Missed and delayed diagnosis of dementia in primary care: prevalence and contributing factors. *Alzheimer Dis Assoc Disord* 2009;23:306–14.

[12] Hinton L, Franz CE, Reddy G, Flores Y, Kravitz RL, Barker JC. Practice constraints, behavioral problems, and dementia care: primary care physicians' perspectives. *J Gen Intern Med* 2007;22:1487–92.

[13] Pimlott NJG, Persaud M, Drummond N, et al. Family physicians and dementia in Canada. Part 2. Understanding the challenges of dementia care. *Can Fam Physician* 2009;55:508–9.e1-7.

[14] Ganguli M, Rodriguez E, Mulsant B, et al. Detection and management of cognitive impairment in primary care: the Steel Valley seniors survey. *J Am Geriatr Soc* 2004;52:1668–75.

[15] Turner S, Iliffe S, Downs M, Wilcock J, et al. General practitioners' knowledge, confidence and attitudes in the diagnosis and management of dementia. *Age Ageing* 2004;33:461–7.

[16] Iliffe S, Wilcock J. The identification of barriers to the recognition of, and response to, dementia in primary care using a modified focus group approach. *Dementia* 2005;4:73–85.

[17] Foster NL. Barriers to treatment: the unique challenges for physicians providing dementia care. *J Geriatr Psychiatry Neurol* 2001;14:188–98.

[18] Valcour VG, Masaki KH, Curb D, Blanchette PL. The detection of dementia in the primary care setting. *Arch Intern Med* 2000;160:2964–8.

[19] Hutchings D, Vanoli A, McKeith I, Brotherton S, Mcnamee P, Bond J. Cholinesterase inhibitors and Alzheimer's disease: patient, care and professional factors influencing the use of drugs for Alzheimer's disease in the United Kingdom. *Dementia* 2010;9:427–43.

[20] Pimlott NJG, Siegel K, Persaud M, et al. Management of dementia by family physicians in academic settings. *Can Fam Physician* 2006;52:1108–9.

[21] Franz CE, Barker JC, Kim K, et al. When help becomes a hindrance: mental health referral systems as barriers to care for primary care physicians treating patients with Alzheimer's disease. *Am J Geriatr Psychiatry* 2010;18:576–85.

[22] Cantegreil-Kallen I, Turbelin C, Angel P, Flahault A, Rigaud A. Dementia management in France: health care and support services in the community. *Dementia* 2006;5:317–26.

[23] Phelan EA, Borson S, Grothaus L, Balch S, Larson EB. Association of incident dementia with hospitalizations. *J Am Med Assoc* 2012;307:165–72.

[24] Burns R, Nichols LO, Martindale-Adams J, Graney MJ, Lummus A. Primary care interventions for dementia caregivers: 2-year outcomes from the REACH study. *Gerontologist* 2003;43:547–55.

[25] Vickrey BG, Mittman BS, Connor KI, et al. The effect of a disease management intervention on quality and outcomes of dementia care: a randomized, controlled trial. *Ann Intern Med* 2006;145:713–26.

[26] Downs M, Turner S, Bryans M, et al. Effectiveness of educational interventions in improving detection and management of dementia in primary care: cluster randomized controlled study. *Br Med J* 2006;332:692–6.

[27] Chodosh J, Berry E, Lee M, et al. Effect of a dementia care management intervention on primary care provider knowledge, attitudes, and perceptions of quality of care. *J Am Geriatr Soc* 2006;54:311–7.

[28] Waldorff FB, Almind G, Makela M, Moller S, Waldemar G. Implementation of a clinical dementia guideline: a controlled study on the effect of a multifaceted strategy. *Scand J Prim Health Care* 2003;21:142–7.

[29] Callahan CM, Boustani MA, Unverzagt FW, et al. Effectiveness of collaborative care for older adults with Alzheimer disease in primary care: a randomized controlled trial. *J Am Med Assoc* 2006;295:2148–57.

[30] Johansson G, Eklund K, Gosman-Hedstrom G. Multidisciplinary team, working with elderly persons living in the community: a systematic literature review. *Scand J Occup Ther* 2010;17:101–16.

[31] Parmar J, Dobbs CB, McKay R, et al. Diagnosis and management of dementia in primary care. *Can Fam Physician* 2014;60:457–65.

[32] Donaldson MS. Continuity of care: a reconceptualization. *Med Care Res Rev* 2001;58:255–90.

[33] Cockerill R, Jaglal S, Charles LL, Chambers L, Brazil K, Cohen C. Components of coordinated care: a new instrument to assess caregivers' and care recipients' experiences with networks of dementia care. *Dementia* 2006;5:51–66.

[34] Prince M, Bryce R, Ferri C. World Alzheimer Report 2011: the benefits of early diagnosis and intervention. *Alzheimer's Disease International: London,* 2011. Available at: www.alz.co.uk/research/world-report. Accessed on April 3, 2014.

[35] Phillips J, Pond D, Goode SM. *Timely Diagnosis of Dementia: Can we do better?* A report for Alzheimer's Australia, 2011. Available at: www.alzheimers.org.au. Accessed on April 3, 2014.

[36] Bamford C, Eccles M, Steen N, Robinson L. Can primary care record review facilitate earlier diagnosis of dementia? *Fam Pract* 2007; 24:108–16.

[37] Pond CD, Brodaty H, Stocks NP, et al. Ageing in general practice (AGP) trial: a cluster randomised trial to examine the effectiveness of peer education on GP diagnostic assessment and management of dementia. *BMC Fam Pract* 2012;13:12.

[38] Justiss MD, Boustani M, Fox C et al. Patients' attitudes of dementia screening across the Atlantic. *Int J Geriatr Psychiatry* 2009; 24:632–7.

[39] Sullivan K, O'Conner F. Should a diagnosis of dementia be disclosed? *Aging Ment Health* 2001;5:340–8.

[40] Banerjee S,Owen J. *Living Well with Dementia: A National Dementia Strategy.* Department of Health: London, 2009.

[41] Edwards R, Voss S and Illife S. Education about dementia in primary care: Is person-centredness the key? *Dementia* 2014;13:111–9.

[42] Downs M, Turner S, Bryans M, et al. Effectiveness of educational interventions in improving detection and management of dementia in primary care: cluster randomised controlled study. *Br Med J* 2006; 332:692–6.

[43] Illife S and Koch T. Tailored education rather than financial incentives are effective educational interventions for primary dementia care. *Int J Geriatr Psychiatry* 2012;27:764–5.

[44] Kennedy A, Reeves D, Bower P, et al. Implementation of self-management support for long-term conditions in routine primary care settings: a cluster randomized controlled trial. *Br Med J* 2013;346:2882.

[45] Schoenmakers B, Buntinx F, Delepeleire J. What is the role of the general practitioner towards the family caregiver of a community-dwelling demented relative? A systematic literature review. *Scand J Prim Health Care 2009;27*:31–40.

[46] Wilkins CH, Wilkins KL, Meisel M, Depke M, Williams J, Edwards DF. Dementia undiagnosed in poor older adults with functional impairment. *J Am Geriatr Soc* 2007;55:1771–6.

[47] Eccles M, Clarke J, Livingstone M, et al. North of England evidence based guidelines development project: guide-line for the primary care management of dementia. *Br Med J* 1998;317:802–8.

[48] Agency for Healthcare Research and Quality. *Recommendations of the U.S. Preventive Services Task Force: Guide to Clinical Preventive Services. AHRQ*: Rockville, MD, 2005. Available at: www.ahrq.gov/clinic/pocketgd.pdf/. Accessed on December 22, 2013.

[49] National Collaborating Centre for Mental Health Dementia: *the NICE/SCIE Guideline on Supporting People with Dementia and Their Carers in Health and Social Care.* National Clinical Practice Guideline 42 and British Psychological Society and Royal College of Psychiatrists: Leicester and London, 2007.

[50] Folstein MF, Bassett SS, Romanoski AJ, Nestadt G. The epidemiology of delirium in the community: The eastern Baltimore mental health. *Int Psychogeriatr* 1991;3:169–76.

[51] Brodaty H, Pond D, Kemp NM, et al. The GPCOG: a new screening test for dementia designed for general practice. *J Am Geriatr Soc* 2002;50:530–4.

[52] Borson S, Scanlan J, Brush M et al. The mini-cog: a cognitive 'vital signs' measure for dementia screening in multi-lingual elderly.. *Int J Geriatr Psychiatry* 2000;15:1021–7.

[53] Buschke H, Kuslansky G, Katz M, et al. Screening for dementia with the Memory Impairment Screen. *Neurology* 1999;52:231–8.

[54] Brooke P, Bullock R. Validation of a 6-item cognitive impairment test with a view to primary care usage. *Int J Geriatr Psychiatry* 1999;14:936–40.

[55] Shulman KI. Clock-drawing: is it the ideal cognitive screening test? *Int J Geriatr Psychiatry* 2000;15:548–61.

[56] *New Recommendations for Detection of Cognitive Impairment During Medicare Annual Wellness Visit.* Available at: http://www.alz.org/professionals_and_researchers_14294.asp#assessvideos. Accessed on May 7, 2013.

[57] Galvin JE, Roe CM, Powlishta KK, et al. The AD8: a brief informant interview to detect dementia. *Neurology*. 2005;65:559–64.

[58] Mitchell AJ, Malladi S. Screening and case finding tools for the detection of dementia. Part I: evidence-based meta-analysis of multidomain tests. *Am J Geriatr Psychiatry* 2010;18:759–82.

[59] Cordell CB, Borson S, Boustani M, et al. Medicare Detection of Cognitive Impairment Workgroup. Alzheimer's Association recommendations for operationalizing the detection of cognitive impairment during the Medicare annual wellness visit in a primary care setting. *Alzheimers Dement*. 2013;9:141–50.

[60] Geldmacher DS, Kerwin DR. Practical Diagnosis and Management of Dementia Due to Alzheimer's Disease in the Primary Care Setting: An Evidence-Based Approach. *Prim Care Companion CNS Disord* 2013;15(4). Published online 2013 Aug 23. Doi: 10.4088:PCC12r Published

[61] Young J, Anstey KJ, Cherbuin N. Online memory screening – are older adults interested and can it work? *Aging Ment Health* 2012;16:931–7.

[62] Dementia Collaborative Research Centre – Assessment and Better Care, University of New South Wales, Sydney, NSW, Australia – The Royal Australian College of General Practitioners (2011). "*14 Essentials for Good Dementia Care in General Practice*". Available at: http://www.dementiaresearch.org.au/. Accessed on April 3, 2014.

[63] Villars H, Oustric S, Andrieu S, et al. The primary care physician and Alzheimer's disease: an international position paper. *J Nutr Health Aging* 2010;14:100–20.

[64] Waldemar G, Dubois B, Emre M, et al. Recommendations for the diagnosis and management of Alzheimer's Disease and other disorders associated with dementia: EFNS guideline. *Eur J Neurol* 2007;14: e1–e26.

[65] Alzheimer's Society. *Diagnosis and Assessment.* Factsheet 426LP Last reviewed: August 2014. Registered charity no. 296645. A company limited by guarantee and registered in England no. 2115499. Available at: http://www.alzheimers.org.uk/. Accessed on April 3, 2015.

[66] Alzheimer's Association. 2011 Alzheimer's disease facts and figures. *Alzheimers Dement* 2011;7:208–44.

[67] Balasa M, Gelpi E, Antonell A, et al. Clinical features and APOE genotype of pathologically proven early-onset Alzheimer disease. *Neurology* 2011;76:1720–5.

[68] Pirani A, Brodaty H, Martini E, Zaccherini D, Neviani F, Neri M. The validation of the Italian version of the GPCOG (GPCOG-It): a contribution to cross-national implementation of a screening test for dementia in general practice. *Int Psychogeriatr* 2010;22:82–90.

[69] Pirani, Brodaty H, Zaccherini D, Tulipani C, Neri M. *A Proposal to Improve Early Diagnosis of Dementia in General Practice*. National Dementia Research Forum: Sydney, Australia, 22–23 September 2011.

[70] Apostolova LG, Cummings JL. Neuropsychiatric manifestations in mild cognitive impairment: a systematic review of the literature. *Dement Geriatr Cogn Disord* 2008;25:115–26.

[71] Boustani MA, Sachs GA, Alder CA, et al. Implementing innovative models of dementia care: the healthy aging brain center. *Aging Ment Health* 2011;15:13–22.

[72] Callahan CM, Boustani MA, Weiner M, et al. Implementing dementia care models in primary care settings: The Aging Brain Care Medical Home. *Aging Ment Health* 2011;15:5–12.

[73] Low L-F, Fletcher J. Models of home care services for people with dementia: a narrative review. *Int Psychogeriatr* 2015;12:1–8.

[74] Moniz-Cook E, Vernooij Dassen M, Woods B, et al. Psychosocial interventions in dementia care research: the INTERDEM manifesto. *Aging Ment Health* 2011;15:283–90.

[75] Smits CH, de Lange J, Dröes RM, Meiland F, Vernooij-Dassen, Pot Am. Effects of combined intervention programmes for people with dementia living at home and their caregivers: a systematic review. Int J Geriatr Psychiatry 2007;22:1181–23.

[76] Olazarán J, Reisberg B, Clare L, et al. Nonpharmacological therapies in Alzheimer's disease: a systematic review of efficacy. *Dement Geriatr Cogn Disord* 2010;30:161–78.

[77] Robinson L, Iliffe S, Brayne C, et al. Primary care in dementia: 2 long-term care at home: psychosocial interventions, information provision, carer support and case management. *Int J Geriatr Psychiatry* 2010;25:657–64.

[78] Vernooij-Dassen M, Draskovic I, McCleery J, et al. Cognitive reframing for carers of people with dementia. *Cochrane Database Syst Rev* 2011; Nov 9;(11):CD005318.

[79] Spector A, Thorgrimsen L, Woods B, et al. *Making a Difference: An Evidence-Based Group Programme to Offer Cognitive Stimulation Therapy (CST) to People with Dementia*. Hawker Publications: London, 2006.

[80] Woods B, Aguirre E, Spector AE et al. Cognitive stimulation to improve cognitive functioning in people with dementia. *Cochrane Database Syst Rev* 2012; 2:CD005562.

[81] Spector A, Thorgrimsen L, Woods RT, et al. Efficacy of an evidence-based cognitive stimulation therapy programme for people with dementia: randomised controlled trial. *Br J Psychiatry* 2003; 183:248–54.

[82] Bunn F, Goodman C, Sworn K, et al. Psychosocial factors that shape patient and carer experiences of dementia diagnosis and treatment: a systematic review of qualitative studies. *PLOS Medicine* 2012; 9:e1001331.

[83] Clare L, Linden DEJ, Woods RT, et al. Goal-oriented cognitive rehabilitation for people with early-stage Alzheimer disease: a single-blind randomized controlled trial of clinical efficacy. *Am J Geriatr Psychiatry* 2010;18:928–39.

[84] Graff MJ, Vernooij-Dassen MJ, Thijssen M, et al. Effects of community occupational therapy on quality of life, mood, and health status in dementia patients and their caregivers: a randomized controlled trial. *J Gerontol A: Biol Sci Med Sci* 2007;62:1002–9.

[85] Perry M, Draskovic I, Lucassen P, et al. Effects of educational interventions on primary dementia care: a systematic review. *Int J Geriatr Psychiatry* 2011;26:1–11.

[86] Connoly A, Iliffe S, Gaehl S, et al. Quality of care provided to people with dementia: utilisation and quality of the annual review in general practice. *Br J Gen Pract* 2012;62:e91–8.

[87] Vasse E, Moniz-Cook E, Olde Rikkert M, et al. The development of quality indicators to improve psychosocial care in dementia. *Int Psychogeriatr* 2012;24:921–30.

[88] Iliffe S, Wilcock J, Haworth D. Delivering psychosocial interventions for people with dementia in primary care: jobs or skills? *Dementia: Int J Soc Res Pract* 2006;5:327–38.

[89] Hodge S, Doncaster E, Moniz-Cook E, et al. Two sides of the same coin? Patients' and carers' views of UK memory services. *Aging Health* 2013;9:275–80.

[90] World Health Organisation (2008). *Integrated Health Services – What and Why.* Technical Brief No. 1, 2008. Available at http://www.who.int/healthsystems/service_delivery_techbrief1.pdf. Accessed on April 9, 2015.

[91] Maidment ID, Fox C, Boustani M, Katona C. Medication management – the missing link in dementia interventions. *Int J Geriatr Psychiatry* 2012;27:439–42.

[92] Department of Health. *The Use of Antipsychotic Medication for People with Dementia: Time for Action*. Stationary Office: London. Available at: www.dh.gov.uk/en/Publicationsandstatistics/Publications/PublicationsPolicyAndGuidance/DH_108303/. Accessed May 7, 2013.

[93] Smith F, Francis SA, Gray N, Denham M, Graffy J. A multi-centre survey among informal carers who manage medication for older care recipients: problems experienced and development of services. *Health Soc Care Community* 2003;11:138–45.

[94] Maidment ID, Haw C, Stubbs J, et al. Medication errors in older people with mental health problems: a review. *Int J Geriatr Psychiatry* 2008;23:564–73.

[95] Maidment ID, Parmentier H. Medication error in mental health: implications for primary care. *Ment Health Fam Med* 2009;6:203–7.

[96] National Institute of Clinical Excellence. *Falls: assessment and prevention of falls in older people*. NICE: London, 2013. Available at: http://www.guidance.nice.org.uk/CG161/. Accessed on May 7, 2013.

[97] Gill SS, Anderson GM, Fischer HD, et al. Syncope and its consequences in patients with dementia receiving cholinesterase inhibitors: a population-based cohort study. *Arch Intern Med* 2009;169:867–73.

[98] Pimouguet C, Lavaud T, Dartigues J, Helmer C. Dementia case management effectiveness on health care costs and resource utilization: a systematic review of randomized controlled trials. *J Nutr Health Aging* 2010;14(8):669–76.

[99] Mittelman M, Haley W, Clay O, Roth D. Improving caregiver well-being delays nursing home placement of patients with Alzheimer Disease. *Neurology* 2006;67:1592–9.

[100] Chien WT, Lee YM. A disease management program for families of persons in Hong Kong with dementia. *Psychiatr Serv* 2008;59:433–6.

[101] Vickery B, Mittman B, Connor K, et al. The effect of disease management intervention study on quality and outcomes of dementia care. *Ann Intern Med* 2006;145:713–72.

[102] Tam-Tham H, Cepoiu-Martin M, Ronksley P E, Maxwell C J, Hemmelgarn BR. Dementia case management and risk of long-term care placement: a systematic review and meta-analysis. *Int J Geriatr Psychiatry* 2013;28:889–902.

[103] Somme D, Trouve H, Dramé M, Gagnon D, Couturier Y, Saint-Jean, O. Analysis of case management programs for patients with dementia: a systematic review. *Alzheimers Dementia* 2012;8:426–36.

[104] Eloniemi-Sulkava U, Notkola IL, Hentinen M, Kivela SL, Sivenius J, Sulkava R. Effects of supporting community-living demented patients and their caregivers: a randomized trial. *J Am Geriatr Soc* 2001;49:1282–7.

[105] Khanassov V, Vedel I, Pluye P. Case management for dementia in primary health care: a systematic mixed studies review based on the diffusion of innovation model. *J Clin Intervent Aging* 2014;9:915–28.

[106] Béland F, Bergman H, Lebel P, et al. Integrated services for frail elders (SIPA): a trial of a model for Canada. *Can J Aging* 2006;25:5–42.

[107] Chatterji P, Burstein NR, Kidder D, White A. *Evaluation of the Program of All-Inclusive Care for the elderly (PACE) Demonstration: The Impact of PACE on Participants Outcomes*. Abt Associations: Cambridge, MA. 1998.

[108] Fabbo A, Capelli O, De Luca ML, De Vreese LP, et al. A model of integrated care for people with dementia in primary care. *Int J Integr Care*. 2014 (WCIC Conf Suppl) URN:NBN:NL:UI:10-1-116641.

[109] Mundt JC, Ferber KL, Greist JH. Symptoms of dementia screener (SDS): treatment and community screening. *Gerontologist.* 2001;41: 131–2.

[110] Patricia PA, et al. Validation of the Cumulative Illness Rating Scale in a geriatric residential population. *J Am Geriatr Soc* 1995; 43.2:130–7.

[111] Graf, C. The Lawton instrumental activities of daily living scale. *Am J Nurs* 2008;108(4):52–62.

[112] Katz S, et al. Studies of illness in the aged: the index of ADL: a standardized measure of biological and psychosocial function. *JAMA* 1963;185:914–9.

[113] First MB. *Structured Clinical Interview for DSM-IV-TR Axis I Disorders: Patient Edition.* Biometrics Research Department, Columbia University, 2005.

[114] Mulhausen P, Chun A, Green A,et al. American Geriatrics Society identifies five things that healthcare providers and patients should question. *J Am Geriatr Soc* 2013;6:622–31.

[115] Chun A, Green A, Hayward A, et al. American Geriatrics Society identifies another five things that healthcare providers and patients should question. *J Am Geriatr Soc* 2014;62:950–60.

[116] Johnston B. *Delirium in the Elderly*. Primary Care Geriatric Lectures, University of California. Available at https://www.coursehero.com/file/6643602/sfdelirium/. Accessed on April 9, 2015.

[117] Inouye S. A multicomponent intervention to prevent delirium in hospitalized older patients. *Ann Intern Med* 1993;119–474.

[118] Ungar A, Salti F, Di Bari M, Di Iorio A. Linee Guida sull'ipertensione arteriosa nell'anziano [Guidelines for hypertension in the elderly]. *G Gerontol* 2000;48:197–203.

[119] Gillespie D, Robertson M, Gillespie J, et al. Interventions for preventing falls in older people living in the community. Editorial Group: Cochrane Bone, Joint and Muscle Trauma Group. Published Online: September 12, 2012. Available at http://onlinelibrary.wiley.com/doi/10.1002/14651858.CD007146.pub3/. Accessed on April 3, 2015.

[120] Musini VM, Tejani AM, Bassett K, Wright JM. Pharmacotherapy for hypertension in the elderly. *Cochrane Database Syst Rev.* 2009;7(4):CD000028.

[121] Cummings JL, Mega M., Gray K, et al. The Neuropychiatric Inventory: a comprehensive assessment of psychopatology in dementia. *Neurology*, 1994;44:2308–14.

[122] Warden V, Hurley AC, Volicer L. Development and psychometric evaluation of the pain assessment in advanced dementia (PAINAD) scale. *J Am Med Dir Assoc* 2003;4:9–15.

[123] Sentagen EA, King SA. The problems of pain and its detection among geriatric nursing home residents. *J Am Geriatr Soc* 1993;41:541–4.

Chapter 5

Cardiovascular Risk Assessment in People Affected with Diabetes in Primary Care

Lucia Borsari, Monica Lorenzini, Silvia Riccomi, Valentina Solfrini,
Marco Vinceti and Oreste Capelli

Additional information is available at the end of the chapter

http://dx.doi.org/10.5772/62646

Abstract

Several studies suggest that the cardiovascular disease (CVD) mortality rates of persons with type 2 diabetes are about two to four times higher than those of the general population. It is therefore considered necessary to develop specific tools to evaluate and reduce CVD risk in this population. In the present chapter, main CVD risk scores were explored: from the Framingham study developed in the 1960s to the last diabetes-specific models, passing through the concept of diabetes as a "CVD risk equivalent". The scores developed in Italian population were specifically explored. The Italian experience, according to other countries, emphasizes that it may be appropriate for each country to validate existing models and eventually to adapt them to the different settings to improve targeted risk management.

Keywords: cardiovascular disease, diabetes mellitus, general practice, primary care, risk models, cardiovascular risk assessment

1. Introduction

Persons with type 2 diabetes are at increased risk for the development of cardiovascular events. Several studies suggest that cardiovascular disease (CVD) is the predominant source of morbidity and early mortality among these patients, with mortality rates about two to four times higher in persons affected with diabetes compared with the general population [1–3]. In particular, a recent study involving almost 1.2 million participants observed a hazard ratio (HR) for mortality of about 2 in patients who suffered from diabetes or myocardial infarction or stroke, while it almost doubles for a combination of CVDs and diabetes [4]. These results

INTECH
open science | open minds

© 2016 The Author(s). Licensee InTech. This chapter is distributed under the terms of the Creative Commons Attribution License (http://creativecommons.org/licenses/by/3.0), which permits unrestricted use, distribution, and reproduction in any medium, provided the original work is properly cited.

emphasize the need to improve CVD preventive strategies specifically oriented to the diabetic population.

1.1. Rationale for CVD risk prediction in people with diabetes

Estimates of CVD risk can be useful for both clinicians and patients: for clinicians, it is a prognostic information that can support them in the choice of therapeutic and preventive strategies; and for patients, it can be a motivation tool to adopt healthy lifestyle measures and to observe prescribed risk-modifying treatments [5].

Considering that diabetes mellitus usually involves the coexistence of several cardiovascular risk factors, it was considered necessary to develop multifactorial approaches for CVD risk evaluation. The first studies aiming at developing reliable tools for evaluating CVD risk based on a combination of several risk factors were carried out in the United States by the Framingham investigators in the 1960s [6]. The Framingham risk score was first developed based on a long-term community cohort study, and it is applicable to general population. One of the main limitations of this model was that it did not consider diabetes status or any other indicator of chronic hyperglycaemia. In the following years, diabetes status was added to the model but only as categorical variable, and the tool was validated only in the general population [7, 8].

Three decades later, in the late 1990s, a study from Finland suggested for the first time that people suffering from diabetes, but without history of CVD, had a risk of CVD similar to that of people without diabetes who had survived a CVD event. Following this observation, several studies supported this concept of diabetes as a "CVD risk equivalent": the presence of diabetes mellitus is considered to confer a 10-year CVD risk similar to individuals without diabetes with a prior history of CVD [9–12]. This approach has been confirmed by algorithms currently developed from both American and European cohorts, such as ATP-III guidelines [13], the European Systematic COronary Risk Evaluation (SCORE) algorithm [14] and the Prospective Cardiovascular Munster (PROCAM) model [15]. In these models, all patients with diabetes mellitus as those with existing CVD are considered as people at high risk and treated as if they required secondary prevention of CVD. In recent years, this approach has been called into question by several authors [16] considering more appropriate to develop diabetes-specific risk models. To date, some authors support the need to create models exclusively from cohorts of persons affected with diabetes, while others prefer to adapt existing risk models developed in the general population to diabetes [17].

2. Overview of diabetes-specific cardiovascular risk models

In contrast to the approach that every patient with diabetes has the same high risk for CVD events, some current guidelines include different treatment recommendations for diabetic patients without other CVD risk factors, who are considered to be at lower risk [18, 19]. In particular, a recent evidence showed a wide distribution of risk in diabetic population depending on, among others, glycated haemoglobin (HbA1c) level and numerous concomitant risk factors [20]. An accurate cardiovascular risk stratification is important in patients with diabetes, as for general population, to determine the type and the intensity of treatment. In a recent systematic review [21], 45 cardiovascular prediction models applicable to patients with diabetes have been identified, of which 12 were specifically designed for patients with type 2 diabetes. Only few of these prediction models were evaluated in independent patient populations.

2.1. The UK Prospective Diabetes Study (UKPDS) risk engine

The oldest and most commonly used prediction model is the UK Prospective Diabetes Study (UKPDS) risk engine. The score was initially designed to estimate coronary heart disease (CHD) risk and stroke risk separately. It was developed on a cohort of 5102 patients with type 2 diabetes followed for a median of 10.7 years [22]. On the contrary, the Framingham calculator that tended to underestimate risks for people with diabetes included relatively few diabetic subjects; it was created using data from 5573 individuals followed for 12 years, but only 337 were known to have diabetes. Moreover, this and the other models for CVD risk evaluation in general population used dichotomous variables for glycaemia, such as the presence or absence of diabetes. The UKPDS diabetes-specific approach included HbA1c as a continuous variable for the first time; it also replaced age as a risk factor by two diabetes-specific variables: age at diagnosis of diabetes and time since the diagnosis of diabetes. Risk factors included in the first UKPDS model and the main limitations of this equation are shown in Table 1.

<table>
<tr><th>Indicators</th><th>Main limitations of the score</th></tr>
<tr><td>Age at diagnosis of diabetes</td><td>It was implemented only in newly diagnosed diabetic patients</td></tr>
<tr><td>Sex</td><td rowspan="5">In may be invalid in specific patient group:
- People outside baseline ranges (25–65 years)
- People diagnosed when <25 years
- People of ethnic background other than Anglo-Celt, Afro-Caribbean or Indian-Asian
- People with prior CVD</td></tr>
<tr><td>Ethnic group</td></tr>
<tr><td>Smoke: current smoking of tobacco in any form, at diagnosis of diabetes</td></tr>
<tr><td>HbA1c (%) mean values</td></tr>
<tr><td>Systolic blood pressure (mmHg), mean values</td></tr>
<tr><td>Total cholesterol/HDL cholesterol ratio, mean values</td><td>It does not consider renal function and diabetic therapy</td></tr>
</table>

Table 1. Risk factors included in the first UKPDS and related limitations

In 2007, a new model was published [23] that estimates CVD risk directly (defined as first occurrence of fatal or non-fatal myocardial infarction, sudden cardiac death, other ischaemic heart disease, fatal or non-fatal stroke, or fatal peripheral vascular disease). The underlying risk equation was first validated in the Collaborative Atorvastatin Diabetes Study (CARDS) cohort, a primary prevention trial including 2838 patients with diabetes [24], and then in the European Prospective Investigation of Cancer (EPIC)-Norfolk Cohort, a prospective cohort study in which patients aged 40–79 years were recruited from general practitioners in the Norfolk region of the United Kingdom [25]. A sample of 10,137 patients, of which 272 diagnosed with diabetes, was extracted from this cohort to evaluate the performance of the UKPDS risk engine compared to the Framingham risk equations in both general and diabetic population. Both these equations performed reasonably well for identifying patients with high CVD risk. UKPDS performed better in diabetic population than the Framingham score, even if both equations overestimated the risk in this group of patients. Considering that in previous studies the Framingham score used in diabetic population underestimated CVD risk [26–29], these tools appear to be very useful to support clinicians in treatment management, but not entirely adequate to communicate risk information to patients.

2.2. Diabetes Audit and Research in Tayside, Scotland (DARTS)

In Tayside, Scotland, a population cohort with type 2 diabetes (4569 men and women of any age) without previous cardiovascular events was constructed from Diabetes Audit and Research in Tayside, Scotland (DARTS) and followed up for a maximum of 9.5 years. Ten risk factors were considered to develop a CVD risk equation, and the main outcome measure for its validation was the first major CHD event (fatal or non-fatal acute myocardial infarction or CHD death) [30].

Compared to UKPDS, the Scottish model has no age restrictions; it includes body mass index (BMI), height, triglycerides and antihypertensive treatment (dichotomous variables: yes/no); and it does not take into account the racial/ethnic background.

2.3. The Action in Diabetes and Vascular disease: preterAx and diamicroN-MR Controlled Evaluation (ADVANCE) risk engine

The Framingham and UKPDS CVD risk models have been validated on a large ethnically different sample of patients with diabetes from the "Action in Diabetes and Vascular disease: preterAx and diamicroN-MR Controlled Evaluation (ADVANCE)" cohort study [31]. The cohort was composed of 7168 persons with diabetes without previous CVD. This validation study revealed that the 4-year absolute risk of CVD events was overestimated by both these models. A new model for risk prediction was consequently assessed to improve performance in a multiethnic cohort of patients. Ten risk factors were included in the ADVANCE risk model: age at diagnosis, gender, duration of diabetes, pulse pressure, retinopathy, atrial fibrillation, HbA1c, log of urinary albumin/creatinine ratio, cholesterol and treated hypertension. The new elements introduced in this model were the attention to comorbidities (retinopathy and atrial fibrillation) and the publication of both a risk-scoring chart [32] and an online calculator [33] to facilitate the uptake of the model in clinical practice.

2.4. The Fremantle Australian risk score

In 2009, a study was published that was conducted on a cohort of CVD-free type 2 diabetes from the Fremantle Diabetes Study (FDS) in Australia, assessing the performance of UKPDS and Framingham scores in the prediction of 5-year CVD [34]. Both these algorithms did not perform satisfactorily in this Australian population. The investigators decided to develop and validate a multivariate risk function for 5-year cardiovascular risk prediction in these patients [35]. A total of 1240 patients with type 2 diabetes were followed from baseline (1993–1996) for

http://dx.doi.org/10.5772/62646

5 years or until they experienced a cardiovascular event or died. CVD during follow-up was defined as hospitalization for myocardial infarction or stroke and death from cardiac or cerebrovascular causes or sudden death. The model includes several variables routinely available in primary care: age, sex, racial/ethnic background (in particular, Aboriginal or Southern-Europe) prior CVD, diabetes treatment (diet, oral hypoglycaemic agents, insulin), serum high-density lipoprotein cholesterol (HDL), HbA1c, urinary albumin (creatinine ratio, mg/mmol) and estimated glomerular filtration rate. Compared to UKPDS, the Australian model includes people with diabetes with prior CVD, it takes into account the racial/ethnic background, it does not consider age at diagnosis and diabetic duration but only current age, and it excludes systolic blood pressure or antihypertensive treatment.

2.5. The New Zealand Diabetes Cohort Study

The New Zealand model for CVD risk assessment in people with diabetes was implemented from the Diabetes Cohort Study (DCS), a prospective open cohort created from a national primary care annual review programme. A total of 36,127 patients with type 2 diabetes without previous CVD was considered to derive a CVD equation. Risk factors taken into account were as follows: age at diagnosis, diabetes duration, sex, systolic blood pressure, smoking status, total cholesterol-to-HDL ratio, ethnicity, HbA1c and urine albumin-to-creatinine ratio. One of the most important characteristics of this model is that was assessed on a very large cohort of patients with diabetes available, thanks to the use of routinely collected data. The authors highlighted the importance of taking into account the ethnicity as a risk factor, which is considered a critical point to reduce health inequalities [36].

2.6. The Swedish National Diabetes Register

The Swedish National Diabetes Register was used to produce a prediction equation for five-year CVD risk in the Swedish diabetic population. The study was based on 11,646 female and male patients, aged 18–70 years. Risk factors considered in this longitudinal study were as follows: age at onset of diabetes, duration of diabetes, HbA1c, BMI, systolic blood pressure, sex, antihypertensive and lipid-lowering drugs and smoking habit [37]. An interesting indicator used in this score is treatment with lipid-lowering drugs, and the main limitation is that it did not include renal function. As for the New Zealand model, the use of routinely collected data, in this case a Disease Register, allowed to include a very large number of patients with diabetes.

3. European Guidelines on Cardiovascular Disease Prevention in Clinical Practice

The latest Guidelines of the European Society of Cardiology (ESC) on CVD Prevention in Clinical Practice [38] recommend total risk estimation using multiple risk factors, such as the SCORE [39], a validated system of risk estimation adopted since the 2003 edition of the above-mentioned guidelines, for asymptomatic adults without evidence of CVD [40]. Moreover, other recommendations are that high-risk individuals can be detected based on established CVD, diabetes mellitus, moderate to severe renal disease, very high levels of individual risk factors or a high SCORE risk, and they are a high priority for intensive advice about all risk factors. However, always in the European context, the recent updates of the guidelines on lipid modification and cardiovascular risk assessment of the National Institute for Health and Care Excellence (NICE) in the United Kingdom [41] recommend the use of a new tool for assessing CVD risk in primary prevention until the age of 84 years and also for persons with type 2 diabetes: the QRISK2 [42].

3.1. QRISK and QRISK2 score

QRISK2 is the development of a previous score, QRISK [43]; the QRISK study, built based on collected from general practice in the United Kingdom, aimed to develop a new algorithm to estimate 10-year risk of CVD (cardiac or cerebrovascular) and to validate its performance against the Framingham and Scottish Score (ASSIGN) algorithms. The derivation cohort of QRISK consisted of persons free of diabetes and existing CVDs. QRISK2, instead, was based on an open cohort of 2.29 million patients (sum of derivation and validation cohort) from UK practices and belonging to different ethnic groups. The cohort was enrolled between 1993 and 2008 with a mean follow-up of 7.3 years for women and 6.9 for men; the considered subjects were aged 32–74 years, without previous recorded diagnosis of CVD and not taking statins at baseline. Many risk factors, such as diabetes, ethnicity and deprivation, are incorporated in the score, which is annually updated and refined (Table 2). A 2011 study for independent and external validation of an updated version of QRISK2 [44] extended the age for risk evaluation and demonstrates good discriminative and calibration properties when compared with the Framingham equation.

QRISK2 Risk factors	
Self-assessed ethnicity	Chronic kidney disease
Age (25–84 years)	Atrial fibrillation
Sex	Systolic blood pressure
UK postcode	Blood pressure treatment
Smoking status	Rheumatoid arthritis
Diabetes status (type 1, type 2 or none)	Ratio of total serum cholesterol/HDL
Family history of coronary heart disease in first-degree relative under 60 years	Body mass index

Table 2. Risk factors: QRISK2 variables included in the web calculator, version 2014 (www.qrisk.org)

Differently from previous editions, the above-mentioned NICE guidelines recommend the use of QRISK2 score also for persons with type 2 diabetes, but not for persons with type 1 diabetes.

http://dx.doi.org/10.5772/62646

The authors validated the QRISK2-2014 version, which collected also the type of diabetes, on a cohort of patients with diabetes (both type 1 and type 2) for the next release of the score in patients with diabetes [45]. In this study, there was no significant improvement for a model that included HbA1c and duration of diabetes, and QRISK-2014 demonstrates to be appropriate for both patients with type 1 and type 2 diabetes. The latest version of QRISK2 (2015) is available at website www.qrisk.org.

3.2. SCORE charts

The SCORE Project assembled a pool of datasets from 12 European cohort studies (205,178 persons), and absolute risk charts (available from website www.escardio.org) were developed separately for high-risk and low-risk regions of Europe. In addition, relative risk charts were developed, helpful for young person with a low absolute but high relative risk, to convey the message of the need for lifestyle change.

An electronic, interactive and improved version of SCORE (available from www.heartscore.org) was also implemented, which is used to accommodate the results of new SCORE analyses, such as those relating to HDL cholesterol, that proved to contribute substantially to risk estimation if entered as an independent variable.

These tools are applicable in primary prevention, and they estimate the 10-year risk of fatal cardiovascular event; the variables used in the model are listed in Table 3, comparing SCORE charts and CUORE project. CVD mortality charts have also been recalibrated for some European countries. According to the European guidelines, the intensity of advice should increase with increasing risk. In general, persons with a CVD risk of ≥5% qualify for intensive advice and may benefit from drug treatment. At risk levels >10%, drug treatment is more frequently required. In subjects older than 60 years, however, these thresholds should be interpreted less strictly, because their age-specific risk is normally around these levels even in the absence of diabetes.

SCORE	CUORE
SCORE model estimates the 10-year risk of fatal cardiovascular event in primary prevention	CUORE model estimates the 10-year risk of fatal and non-fatal cardiovascular event in primary prevention
Age (more detailed in 50–65 age range. Charts provided for 40–65 years)	Age (40–69 years for charts, 35–69 years for individual score)
Sex	Sex
Systolic blood pressure	Systolic blood pressure
–	Antihypertensive treatment (only for individual score)
Total cholesterol	Total cholesterol
HDL cholesterol	HDL cholesterol (only for individual score)
Smoking habits	Smoking habits
–	Diabetes

Table 3. Risk factors included in SCORE and CUORE projects

4. Cardiovascular risk assessment models in Italy: from individual's global risk evaluation to diabetes-specific models

4.1. The CUORE Project

The Italian version of CVD Prevention Guidelines [18] stated that for Italy it is preferable to use the tools of CUORE Project of the National Institute of Health to estimate CVD risk in the general population. Several studies on Italian cohorts have compared SCORE and CUORE tools: a study published in 2010 [46] highlighted that the first one reflects quite well the Italian cardiovascular mortality, and, correspondingly, Italian cohorts of CUORE Project are quite representative of European countries with a low risk of cardiovascular mortality, at least as regards male subjects. It was not possible to make the same evaluation for women, because the number of fatal cardiovascular events was not enough to allow a reliable estimate of the risk functions. Other studies found moderate level of agreement between the two tools, in particular in discriminating high-risk subjects. The reasons may be attributed in one case to the use of a smaller and different sample of cases than the previous study [47] and in the other case to the "threshold issue" in the score [48]; in this last study, in fact, using risk scores as continuous variables, the concordance between SCORE and CUORE tools resulted higher.

Since 1998, the year of its birth, the CUORE Project aimed at the following objectives [49]:

- to implement a population-based register of cardiovascular events;
- to realize a survey to assess risk factors distribution, prevalence of high-risk conditions and CVD;
- to assess cardiovascular risk of the Italian population and make tools for risk assessment easily applicable;
- to implement a training plan on cardiovascular risk assessment for General Practitioners;
- to explain the declining trend of mortality for CHDs; and
- to update the Italian tools for risk prediction.

The global cardiovascular risk score of CUORE Project was developed using data from different cohorts enrolled in the north, centre and south of Italy between the 1980s and the 1990s, whose risk factors had been collected using standardized procedures. It was validated on 20,647 persons, with a median follow-up duration of 9.5 years for men and 8.0 years for women [50]. The individual score (available from website www.cuore.iss.it) can be calculated in subjects aged 35–69 years and predicts 10-year risk of a first fatal and non-fatal cardiovascular event based on risk factors listed in Table 3. In addition to the individual score, are also available risk charts, which differ for the number of risk factors used and for the age group in which they are applied (Table 3) and moreover for accuracy of information (charts are less accurate, offering classes of absolute global risk calculated for categories of risk factors). According to this tool, individuals are considered at high risk if their 10-year CVD risk is 20% or more; instead, they are at low risk if it is <5%; risk categories were stratified in six levels.

As shown in Table 3, differently from CUORE Project, SCORE risk charts do not include a dichotomous diabetes variable into the risk function, because there was a lack of uniformity in the ascertainment of diabetes. Furthermore, the instruction for the use of these charts argues that they underestimate the risk in patients with diabetes and should be used only in patients with type 1 diabetes without any target organ damage. It must be emphasized that, as mentioned above, ESC Guidelines on CVD Prevention, also in its versions for diabetes, prediabetes and CVDs [51], ranks subjects with diabetes mellitus (both type 1 and type 2), respectively, at high or very high risk, depending on whether they have one or more cardiovascular risk factors and/or target organ damage.

As concluded by the World Health Organization Multinational Study Group on Vascular Disease in Diabetes, developments in the assessment of CVD risk in diabetes must include diabetes-related variables as well as the conventional risk factors [52].

The Italian "National Prevention Plan" 2005–2007 and 2010–2012 included 10-year cardiovascular risk assessment using the CUORE Project's tools [53], and this allowed the realization of a national training programme for general practitioners. Preliminary results underline the importance of its evaluation in clinical practice and demonstrate the feasibility to implement a risk factor surveillance system involving trained general practitioners [49, 54].

Moreover, guidelines and studies on these issues emphasize the need for updating charts and scores for risk assessment, since population's risk profile and mortality for CVD change over time. It is therefore necessary to enrol new cohorts or to update existing ones. In this perspective, CUORE Project has expanded database of cardiovascular risk factors by adding the cohort of the Osservatorio Epidemiologico Cardiovascolare (OEC), enlisted in the late 1990s and was followed until December 2004. Preliminary analyses have confirmed for both men and women the predictive role of the main risk factors is already included in the algorithm, but additional studies should be conducted to assess the inclusion of new risk factors, primarily glycaemia [55].

4.1.1. Use of cardiovascular risk score for lipid-lowering reimbursement

In the recent past, cardiovascular risk assessment obtained through CUORE Project's tools was scarcely applied, despite recommendations of their use from the Ministry of Health to assess cardiovascular risk for statins reimbursement in primary prevention, laid down in the past version of the Italian Medicines Agency (Agenzia Italiana del Farmaco, AIFA) Note 13. Also data from PASSI Study 2009–2012 [56] found that risk chart is still rarely used: only 7% of interviewed aged 35–69 years, without CVD, said that their CVD risk was measured, with significant differences at regional level. It is, however, likely this is an underestimation, being based on patient's interviews and not on medical records data. Recent updates on Note 13 provide, however, for the use of SCORE charts for lipid-lowering reimbursement by National Health System.

Italian cohorts of the CUORE project are quite representative of the European countries at low risk for cardiovascular mortality, and the > 5% risk of fatal CV events in SCORE charts corresponds to a >20% risk of fatal CV events in CUORE Project. Furthermore, the Italian contribution to the cohort used to define SCORE charts was 6% of the subjects evaluated for men and 8% for women, and the duration of follow-up was higher in CUORE Project. On this basis, about the definition of risk levels, the Multidisciplinary Working Group of the Emilia-Romagna Region Drug Commission reaffirmed the validity of CUORE charts and the possibility to continue using them in clinical practice, with the established conversion between CUORE and SCORE risks [57]. Moreover, the estimation of fatal and non-fatal CV events that characterizes CUORE algorithm also allows a better transfer of clinical trial results.

4.2. The Riskard score

Another tool for cardiovascular risk assessment was developed in Italy. The Research Group for Assessment of Cardiovascular Risk in Italy developed a risk chart [58, 59] and then a software named Riskard 2002 [60]. The study enrolled a cohort of over 9000 individuals from three Italian studies, aged 35–74 years and followed up from 5 to 15 years. In subsequent years, the chart and the software were further updated (Riskard 2005), with the purpose to offer tools based on larger and more diversified populations, larger numbers of individuals exposed to risk and events, longer follow-up periods and some other innovative concepts. The chart, by its nature, can incorporate only a limited number of risk factors, while many more can be included in the software [61]. Data were collected from nine population studies in eight Italian regions, for a total of 17.153 subjects. The new chart that allows an estimate of the 10-year risk of undergoing a first cardiovascular event was produced for men and women aged 45–74 years, free from CVDs. Estimates were produced for absolute risk and for relative risk for CVD, the latter against levels expected in the general population.

The software, instead, was produced to predict risk of major coronary, cerebrovascular and cardiovascular events for follow-up at 5, 10 or 15 years, in men and women aged 35–74 years at entry and free from CVDs. Risk factors taken into consideration in the Riskard 2005 software were sex, age, BMI, mean physiological blood pressure, HDL cholesterol, non-HDL cholesterol, cigarette smoking, diabetes and heart rate. The output yielded several indicators, such as absolute risk, relative risk (as defined above), ideal risk (for a very favourable risk profile) and biological age of risk.

4.3. Cardiovascular risk assessment in cohorts of Italian patients with type 2 diabetes

In a recent systematic review that compared performance of CVD risk models developed exclusively from people with diabetes and those developed in the general population [62], a study conducted in Italy in three diabetes clinics of Modena was also included [63]. The study involved 1532 patients and aimed to evaluate the prognostic accuracy of four algorithms used to estimate cardiovascular risk: the UKPDS (constructed on a population of persons with type 2 diabetes), the Framingham and two Italian algorithms, the Riskard and the CUORE.

The Framingham model shows a risk overestimation in the Italian population; also, the function proposed by the UKPDS study, when applied for Italian diabetic population, tends to overestimate cardiovascular risk, without differences between sexes.

Taking into account the Italian situation, the most widely adopted function, the CUORE Project algorithm, underestimates cardiovascular risk, particularly in females. The Riskard algorithm appears more coherent on the evaluation of cardiovascular risk in the cohort examined; however, dividing population according to sex, an overestimation of events in males and large underestimation in females emerge. So, these algorithms agree in overestimating risk in males and underestimating risk in females.

The conclusions are that estimation of cardiovascular risk is dependent on the algorithm used and on the baseline risk of the reference cohort, and functions designed for a specific population, including risk variables peculiar for diabetes, should be adopted to increase the performance of such functions.

4.4. An Italian score for quality of diabetes care evaluation and its association with cardiovascular event risk

In recent years, the pressure on Health Care Systems to deliver high-quality care while controlling costs progressively increased. In this context, the Qualità ed Esito in Diabetologia (QuED) study was developed [64], whose main aim was to develop a score for evaluating quality of diabetes care. In this study, the close relation between a score of quality of diabetes care and long-term outcomes was documented. The QuED study was conducted in Italy by the Consorzio Mario Negri Sud—Department of Clinical Pharmacology and Epidemiology, in collaboration with the Center for Health Policy Research—University of California, Irvine. Overall, 101 diabetes outpatient clinics and 103 general practitioners from all regions of Italy participated in the study, enrolling, respectively, 2448 and 785 patients with type 2 diabetes irrespective of age, diabetes duration or treatment. These patients, representative of all settings of diabetes care, were recruited from March 1998 and December 1999 and followed up for a median of 5 years. The score was calculated using process and intermediate outcome indicators readily available (HbA1c, blood pressure, low-density lipoprotein cholesterol, microalbuminuria) and consistent with those adopted for other initiatives such as the Diabetes Quality Improvement Project (DQIP) [65], started in 1997 in the United States to implement a comprehensive set of national measures for quality improvement. The only difference was the use of a lower threshold for HbA1c (8%) and the addiction of a process indicator, referring to the use of ACE inhibitors in the presence of microalbuminuria, based on evidence that linked it to cardiovascular risk [66]. In the tool construction, a discrete score was given to each variable as follows: 0 points if the patient was not treated for the specific condition despite elevated values, or the patient showed unsatisfactory values despite the treatment; 5 points if the measurement of a parameter was not performed in the latest 12 months; 10 points if the desired goals were attained. The indicators and cut-off used are shown in Table 4. This score ranged from 0 to 40, with a higher score reflecting better quality of care. This score was defined in the following studies also as Q-Score.

The study shows that the risk to develop a cardiovascular event was 89% greater in patients with a score of ≤10 and 43% higher in those with a score between 10 and 20, when compared to patients with a score of >20. It is also important to emphasize that a linear relation between

Indicators	Cut-off
HbA1c	<8%
Blood pressure	<140–90
LDL cholesterol	<3.37 mmol/L (130 mg/dl)
Microalbuminuria	<30 mg/die or ≥30 mg/die with ACEinhibitors or ARB treatment

Note: ACE = angiotensin-converting enzyme; ARB = angiotensin receptor blocker.

Table 4. Quality-of-care scoring system (QUED and QUASAR studies)

QuED score and incidence of cardiovascular events was documented both in patients with and without previous cardiovascular events, and this was true for different outcomes, such as CHD, cerebrovascular accidents, peripheral vascular disease and cardiovascular mortality. The authors stated that QuED score is not intended to replace other risk models utilized to predict the individual risk of cardiovascular events, but rather an indicator of the average quality of the diabetes care provided by a specific setting in health care system.

On this basis, subsequently, the Italian Associazione Medici Diabetologi (AMD), a scientific society, realized the QUASAR study (Quality Assessment Score and Cardiovascular Outcomes in Italian Diabetes Patients) [67]. The score developed and validated in QuED study was applied to the QUASAR population (5181 patients enrolled in 67 Italian diabetes clinics and followed up for a median of 28 months) and was confirmed the strong correlation between this quality of care score and cardiovascular events, both in patient with and without previous cardiovascular events. In QUASAR study, the risk to develop a new cardiovascular event was 84% higher in patients with a score of <15 and 17% higher in those with a score between 15 and 25, when compared with those with a score of >25. This simple score began to be widely used to monitor quality of care and compare the performance of different diabetes clinics [68]. A further article published by the same working group analysed the trends over 8 years in quality of diabetes care, evaluating process and outcome indicators, indicators of treatment intensity or appropriateness and the score developed in QuED and QUASAR [69]. The studies showed a relevant improvement in quality of care for diabetes in Italy from 2004 to 2011, while the economic resources available did not increase. The authors hypothesized that systematic control of quality of care through regular collection of data improved adherence to standards of care and that longitudinal improvements in Q score can be translated in less cardiovascular events. Along years, an increasing numbers of diabetes clinics participated in the AMD initiatives.

4.4.1. Q-home: the application of Q score to a cohort of people with type 2 diabetes in general practice

In the contest of type 2 diabetes integrated care of Local Health Authority (ASL) of Modena in Italy, Q score has been adopted and transposed by the more special setting to that of general practice and it formed the cornerstone for creating an individual and collective report and for developing audit (Q-home). The involvement of general practitioners by returning data analysis on patients with diabetes through dedicated annual reports and digitization of data collection on individual patients has led, over 3 years, to the involvement of a growing cohort of patients (from about 12.000 to 18.000) and of almost all general practitioner of the Modena AUSL. The rate of missing data was analysed and showed a marked decrease, as shown in Table 5.

Indicators	Missing rate (%)	
	2011	2013
HbA1c	9	5
Blood pressure	11	6
LDL cholesterol	12	9
Microalbuminuria	16	12

Table 5. Missing rate of collected data in Q-home project through 3 years.

In the period of 2011–2013, in parallel, the number of all parameters in range grew. Consequently, the percentual of the population with Q score between 30 and 40 points increased. In 2013, all Health Districts were homogenized with each other and exceeded the threshold of 30 points of mean Q score. The next step of the study group will be to associate individual Q score with annual cardiovascular events, hospitalizations, revascularization, access to the emergency department and deaths from all causes. Five years of observation will be considered (from 2011 to 2015), to validate the Q score in general practice, obtaining percentages of risk specific for this setting.

5. Patient–doctor communication on cardiovascular risk

If, on the one hand, giving cardiovascular risk communication to the patient is not simple, on the other hand, it is not clear what and how much the patient understands about the message received.

To date, few studies have been conducted on this topic, and most of these count few patients surveyed. A low awareness of the disease is highlighted. In particular, patients remain anchored to a conception of diabetes as a glycaemic problem, rather than as a pathology at high cardiovascular risk [70–73]. Among the studies that investigated the perception of risk, in Italy, the PRICAD Study (Percezione del RIschio CArdiovascolare nella popolazione Diabetica), promoted by the Associazione Italiana Medici di Famiglia (AIMEF), is designed for the purpose of trying to measure how the patient perceives the diabetes in the context of cardiovascular risk [73]. More than 11,000 persons were actively encouraged to meet the questionnaire, but only 4600 (41%) answered. The majority of them (60%) said that diabetes is only an excess of glucose in the blood and that it is possible to get old in good health despite diabetes. More than half of the subjects fail to recognize the importance of controlling cardiovascular risk factors and believe to have the same blood pressure, cholesterol and BMI target of a peer without diabetes. Only 9% of respondents, less than a fifth the people asked, expressed a serious concern for the greater complication of diabetes.

Analysing the frequencies of concerns considered higher by persons with diabetes, losing the driving licence emerges as an element of utmost concern, while only 9.3% consider the fear for cardiovascular complications a factor of maximum concern. Only 30% of people with diabetes are aware of the close relation between diabetes and cardiovascular risk. Almost two-thirds of the persons with diabetes believe that their blood pressure and cholesterol goals are similar to those of other hypertensive patients. The same lack of awareness is also common in people without diabetes but having other cardiovascular risk factors [74]. Where available, visual tools of communication were of help for the patient in the understanding of the risk [75–77]. Unfortunately, even among patients who receive a clear illustration of their cardiovascular risk, it is not observed a clear memory of what perceived, neither there is a significant nor lasting permanence in their lifestyle change [78].

6. Conclusions

In the present chapter, the main CVD risk scores for patients with diabetes are explored, starting from the first one developed in the 1960s, the Framingham study, to the latest diabetes-specific models. In recent years, diabetic disease is included in most models, even if only the absence or presence of the disease is considered in most of them. The level of HbA1c or blood glucose seems to be an important indicator for the evaluation of CVD risk in both diabetic and general population, and in particular diabetes-specific scores should take into account these variables. It could be useful also to detect impaired fasting glucose (IFG) and impaired glucose tolerance (IGT) conditions in persons without diabetes and to assess the metabolic balance in persons with diabetes. In general, the most recent studies agree on the importance of using diabetic-specific cohorts to adequately assess CVD risk models in this population. Furthermore, the diabetes care settings and the ethnic group need to be taken into account in the development and evaluation of CVD risk in patients with diabetes. Literature data highlight that cardiovascular risk prediction models perform non-optimally in people with diabetes of different ethnic groups. Thus, it may be appropriate for each country to validate the existing models on their populations and eventually to adapt them to the different setting, to improve targeted risk management.

Risk modelling and stratification are important tools for clinicians, because these models represent a useful guide for therapeutic decisions and for patients monitoring. Furthermore, they can be used to communicate with patients and to improve their compliance. In this regard, new strategies are needed to optimize patient's understanding and the internalization of its own level of risk.

Author details

Lucia Borsari[1*], Monica Lorenzini[2], Silvia Riccomi[3], Valentina Solfrini[2], Marco Vinceti[1] and Oreste Capelli[2]

*Address all correspondence to: lucia.borsari@unimore.it; lucybors@hotmail.it

1 Department of Biomedical, Metabolic and Neural Sciences, University of Modena and Reggio Emilia, Modena, Italy

2 Clinical Governance, Local Health Authority of Modena, Modena, Italy

3 Local Health Authority of Modena, Modena, Italy

References

[1] Emerging Risk Factors Collaboration, Sarwar N, Gao P, Seshasai SRK, Gobin R, Kaptoge S, et al. Diabetes mellitus, fasting blood glucose concentration, and risk of vascular disease: a collaborative meta-analysis of 102 prospective studies. Lancet 2010;375(9733):2215–22.

[2] Haffner SM, Lehto S, Rönnemaa T, Pyörälä K, Laakso M. Mortality from coronary heart disease in subjects with type 2 diabetes and in nondiabetic subjects with and without prior myocardial infarction. N Engl J Med. 1998;339(4):229–34.

[3] Gu K, Cowie CC, Harris MI. Mortality in adults with and without diabetes in a national cohort of the U.S. population, 1971–1993. Diabetes Care 1998;21(7):1138–45.

[4] Emerging Risk Factors Collaboration, Di Angelantonio E, Kaptoge S, Wormser D, Willeit P, et al. Association of cardiometabolic multimorbidity with mortality. JAMA 2015;314(1):52–60.

[5] Moons KGM, Kengne AP, Grobbee DE, Royston P, Vergouwe Y, Altman DG, et al. Risk prediction models: II. External validation, model updating, and impact assessment. Heart Br Card Soc. 2012;98(9):691–8.

[6] Truett J, Cornfield J, Kannel W. A multivariate analysis of the risk of coronary heart disease in Framingham. J Chronic Dis. 1967;20(7):511–24.

[7] Ramachandran S, French JM, Vanderpump MP, Croft P, Neary RH. Using the Framingham model to predict heart disease in the United Kingdom: retrospective study. BMJ 2000;320(7236):676–7.

[8] D'Agostino RB, Grundy S, Sullivan LM, Wilson P, CHD Risk Prediction Group. Validation of the Framingham coronary heart disease prediction scores: results of a multiple ethnic groups investigation. JAMA 2001;286(2):180–7.

[9] Wilson PW, D'Agostino RB, Levy D, Belanger AM, Silbershatz H, Kannel WB. Prediction of coronary heart disease using risk factor categories. Circulation 1998;97(18): 1837–47.

[10] Haffner SM, Lehto S, Rönnemaa T, Pyörälä K, Laakso M. Mortality from coronary heart disease in subjects with type 2 diabetes and in nondiabetic subjects with and without prior myocardial infarction. N Engl J Med. 1998;339(4):229–34.

[11] Evans JMM, Wang J, Morris AD. Comparison of cardiovascular risk between patients with type 2 diabetes and those who had had a myocardial infarction: cross sectional and cohort studies. BMJ 2002;324(7343):939–42.

[12] Eberly LE, Cohen JD, Prineas R, Yang L, Intervention Trial Research Group. Impact of incident diabetes and incident nonfatal cardiovascular disease on 18-year mortality: the multiple risk factor intervention trial experience. Diabetes Care 2003;26(3): 848–54.

[13] National Cholesterol Education Program (NCEP) Expert Panel on Detection, Evaluation, and Treatment of High Blood Cholesterol in Adults (Adult Treatment Panel III). Third Report of the National Cholesterol Education Program (NCEP) Expert Panel on Detection, Evaluation, and Treatment of High Blood Cholesterol in Adults (Adult Treatment Panel III) final report. Circulation 2002;106(25):3143–421.

[14] Conroy RM, Pyörälä K, Fitzgerald AP, Sans S, Menotti A, De Backer G, et al. Estimation of ten-year risk of fatal cardiovascular disease in Europe: the SCORE project. Eur Heart J. 2003;24(11):987–1003.

[15] Assmann G, Cullen P, Schulte H. Simple scoring scheme for calculating the risk of acute coronary events based on the 10-year follow-up of the prospective cardiovascular Münster (PROCAM) study. Circulation 2002;105(3):310–5.

[16] Bulugahapitiya U, Siyambalapitiya S, Sithole J, Idris I. Is diabetes a coronary risk equivalent? Systematic review and meta-analysis. Diabet Med J Br Diabet Assoc. 2009;26(2):142–8.

[17] Van Dieren S, Beulens JWJ, Kengne AP, Peelen LM, Rutten GEHM, Woodward M, et al. Prediction models for the risk of cardiovascular disease in patients with type 2 diabetes: a systematic review. Heart Br Card Soc. 2012;98(5):360–9.

[18] Perk J, De Backer G, Gohlke H, Graham I, Reiner Z, Verschuren WMM, et al. European Guidelines on Cardiovascular Disease Prevention in Clinical Practice (version 2012). The Fifth Joint Task Force of the European Society of Cardiology and other societies on cardiovascular disease prevention in clinical practice (constituted by representatives of nine societies and by invited experts). G Ital Cardiol. 2013;14(5):328–92.

[19] American Diabetes Association. Standards of medical care in diabetes – 2013. Diabetes Care 2013;36(Suppl. 1):S11–66.

[20] Howard BV, Best LG, Galloway JM, Howard WJ, Jones K, Lee ET, et al. Coronary heart disease risk equivalence in diabetes depends on concomitant risk factors. Diabetes Care 2006;29(2):391–7.

[21] Van Dieren S, Beulens JWJ, Kengne AP, Peelen LM, Rutten GEHM, Woodward M, et al. Prediction models for the risk of cardiovascular disease in patients with type 2 diabetes: a systematic review. Heart Br Card Soc. 2012;98(5):360–9.

[22] Stevens RJ, Kothari V, Adler AI, Stratton IM, United Kingdom Prospective Diabetes Study (UKPDS) Group. The UKPDS risk engine: a model for the risk of coronary heart disease in Type II diabetes (UKPDS 56). Clin Sci Lond Engl. 2001;101(6):671–9.

[23] Coleman R, Stevens R, Holman R. The Oxford Risk Engine: a cardiovascular risk calculator for individuals with or without type 2 diabetes. Diabetes 2007;56(Suppl. 1):A170.

[24] Mount Hood 4 Modeling Group. Computer modeling of diabetes and its complications: a report on the Fourth Mount Hood Challenge Meeting. Diabetes Care 2007;30(6):1638–46.

[25] Day N, Oakes S, Luben R, Khaw KT, Bingham S, Welch A, et al. EPIC-Norfolk: study design and characteristics of the cohort. European Prospective Investigation of Cancer. Br J Cancer. 1999;80(Suppl. 1):95–103.

[26] McEwan P, Williams JE, Griffiths JD, Bagust A, Peters JR, Hopkinson P, et al. Evaluating the performance of the Framingham risk equations in a population with diabetes. Diabet Med J Br Diabet Assoc. 2004;21(4):318–23.

[27] Yeo WW, Yeo KR. Predicting CHD risk in patients with diabetes mellitus. Diabet Med J Br Diabet Assoc. 2001;18(5):341–4.

[28] Stevens RJ, Coleman RL, Holman RR. Framingham risk equations underestimate coronary heart disease risk in diabetes. Diabet Med J Br Diabet Assoc. 2005;22(2):228.

[29] Guzder RN, Gatling W, Mullee MA, Mehta RL, Byrne CD. Prognostic value of the Framingham cardiovascular risk equation and the UKPDS risk engine for coronary heart disease in newly diagnosed Type 2 diabetes: results from a United Kingdom study. Diabet Med J Br Diabet Assoc. 2005;22(5):554–62.

[30] Donnan PT, Donnelly L, New JP, Morris AD. Derivation and validation of a prediction score for major coronary heart disease events in a U.K. type 2 diabetic population. Diabetes Care 2006;29(6):1231–6.

[31] Kengne AP. The ADVANCE cardiovascular risk model and current strategies for cardiovascular disease risk evaluation in people with diabetes. Cardiovasc J Afr. 2013;24(9–10):376–81.

[32] Kengne AP, Patel A, Marre M, Travert F, Lievre M, Zoungas S, et al. Contemporary model for cardiovascular risk prediction in people with type 2 diabetes. Eur J Cardio-

vasc Prev Rehabil Off J Eur Soc Cardiol Work Groups Epidemiol Prev Card Rehabil Exerc Physiol. 2011;18(3):393–8.

[33] The ADVANCE Collaborative Group. ADVANCE Risk Engine. Available from http://www.advanceriskengine.com/index.html [Accessed April 9, 2015].

[34] Davis WA, Colagiuri S, Davis TME. Comparison of the Framingham and United Kingdom Prospective Diabetes Study cardiovascular risk equations in Australian patients with type 2 diabetes from the Fremantle Diabetes Study. Med J Aust. 2009;190(4):180–4.

[35] Davis WA, Knuiman MW, Davis TME. An Australian cardiovascular risk equation for type 2 diabetes: the Fremantle Diabetes Study. Intern Med J. 2010;40(4):286–92.

[36] Elley CR, Robinson E, Kenealy T, Bramley D, Drury PL. Derivation and validation of a new cardiovascular risk score for people with type 2 diabetes: the New Zealand Diabetes Cohort Study. Diabetes Care 2010;33(6):1347–52.

[37] Cederholm J, Eeg-Olofsson K, Eliasson B, Zethelius B, Nilsson PM, Gudbjörnsdottir S, et al. Risk prediction of cardiovascular disease in type 2 diabetes: a risk equation from the Swedish National Diabetes Register. Diabetes Care 2008;31(10):2038–43.

[38] Fifth Joint Task Force of the European Society of Cardiology, European Association of Echocardiography, European Association of Percutaneous Cardiovascular Interventions, European Heart Rhythm Association, Heart Failure Association, European Association for Cardiovascular Prevention & Rehabilitation, et al. European Guidelines on cardiovascular disease prevention in clinical practice (version 2012): the Fifth Joint Task Force of the European Society of Cardiology and Other Societies on Cardiovascular Disease Prevention in Clinical Practice (constituted by representatives of nine societies and by invited experts). Eur J Prev Cardiol. 2012;19(4):585–667.

[39] Conroy RM, Pyörälä K, Fitzgerald AP, Sans S, Menotti A, De Backer G, et al. Estimation of ten-year risk of fatal cardiovascular disease in Europe: the SCORE project. Eur Heart J. 2003;24(11):987–1003.

[40] De Backer G, Ambrosioni E, Borch-Johnsen K, Brotons C, Cifkova R, Dallongeville J, et al. European guidelines on cardiovascular disease prevention in clinical practice: Third Joint Task Force of European and Other Societies on Cardiovascular Disease Prevention in Clinical Practice (constituted by representatives of eight societies and by invited experts). Eur J Cardiovasc Prev Rehabil Off J Eur Soc Cardiol Work Groups Epidemiol Prev Card Rehabil Exerc Physiol. 2003;10(4):S1–10.

[41] National Clinical Guideline Centre (UK). Lipid Modification: Cardiovascular Risk Assessment and the Modification of Blood Lipids for the Primary and Secondary Prevention of Cardiovascular Disease. London: National Institute for Health and Care Excellence (UK), 2015. Available from guidance.nice.org.uk/cg181 [Accessed April 22, 2015].

[42] Hippisley-Cox J, Coupland C, Vinogradova Y, Robson J, Minhas R, Sheikh A, et al. Predicting cardiovascular risk in England and Wales: prospective derivation and validation of QRISK2. BMJ 2008;336(7659):1475–82.

[43] Hippisley-Cox J, Coupland C, Vinogradova Y, Robson J, May M, Brindle P. Derivation and validation of QRISK, a new cardiovascular disease risk score for the United Kingdom: prospective open cohort study. BMJ 2007;335(7611):136.

[44] Collins GS, Altman DG. Predicting the 10 year risk of cardiovascular disease in the United Kingdom: independent and external validation of an updated version of QRISK2. BMJ 2012;344:4181.

[45] Hippisley-Cox J, Coupland CA, Brindle P. Validation of QRISK2 (2014) in patients with diabetes. Available from www.qrisk.org [accessed April 22, 2015].

[46] Donfrancesco C, Palmieri L, Vanuzzo D, Panico S, Cesana G, Ferrario M, et al. Italian cardiovascular mortality charts of the CUORE Project: are they comparable with the SCORE charts? G Ital Cardiol. 2010;11(2):148–53.

[47] Giavarina D, Barzon E, Cigolini M, Mezzena G, Soffiati G. Comparison of methods to identify individuals at increased risk of cardiovascular disease in Italian cohorts. Nutr Metab Cardiovasc Dis NMCD. 2007;17(4):311–8.

[48] Manzoli L, Palumbo W, Ruotolo P, Panella M, Mezzetti A, Di Stanislao F. Cardiovascular risk of the general population assessed through SCORE and CUORE charts: an extensive survey by the General Practitioners from Abruzzo, Italy. Int J Cardiol. 2010;144(1):47–52.

[49] Palmieri L, Donfrancesco C, Lo Noce C, Dima F, Vannucchi S, Vanuzzo D, Ferrario MM, Cesana G, Panico S, Iacovello L, De Santis Caiola P, Meduri FR, Giampaoli S. Il progetto CUORE: 15 anni di attività per la prevenzione e la riduzione del rischio cardiovascolare. Not Ist Super Sanità. 2013;26(2):3–8.

[50] Palmieri L, Panico S, Vanuzzo D, Ferrario M, Pilotto L, Sega R, et al. Evaluation of the global cardiovascular absolute risk: the Progetto CUORE individual score. Ann Ist Super Sanità. 2004;40(4):393–9.

[51] Authors/Task Force Members, Rydén L, Grant PJ, Anker SD, Berne C, Cosentino F, et al. ESC guidelines on diabetes, pre-diabetes, and cardiovascular diseases developed in collaboration with the EASD: the task force on diabetes, pre-diabetes, and cardiovascular diseases of the European Society of Cardiology (ESC) and developed in collaboration with the European Association for the Study of Diabetes (EASD). Eur Heart J. 2013;34(39):3035–87.

[52] Fuller JH, Stevens LK, Wang SL. Risk factors for cardiovascular mortality and morbidity: the WHO Multinational Study of Vascular Disease in Diabetes. Diabetologia 2001;44(Suppl. 2):S54–64.

[53] Ministry of Health – Italy. National Prevention Plan 2010–2012. Available from www.ccm-network.it [Accessed April 12, 2015].

[54] Palmieri L, Rielli R, Demattè L, Donfrancesco C, Ciccarelli P, De Sanctis Caiola P, et al. CUORE project: implementation of the 10-year risk score. Eur J Cardiovasc Prev Rehabil Off J Eur Soc Cardiol Work Groups Epidemiol Prev Card Rehabil Exerc Physiol. 2011;18(4):642–9.

[55] Donfrancesco C, Palmieri L, Vanuzzo D, Panico S, Ferrario MM, Cesana G, et al. The CUORE Project: preliminary analysis for the updating of the cardiovascular risk charts and individual scores. G Ital Cardiol (Rome). 2010;11(5 Suppl. 3):20S–4S.

[56] National Institute of Health. National Report PASSI 2012: prevention and control of cardiovascular risk. Available from http://www.epicentro.iss.it/passi/rapporto2012/cardiovascolare.asp [Accessed April 8, 2015].

[57] Damiani G, Federico B, Anselmi A, Bianchi CB, Silvestrini G, Iodice L, Navarra P, Da Cas R, Raschetti R, Ricciardi W The impact of regional co-payment and national reimbursement criteria on statins use in Italy: an interrupted time-series analysis. BMC Health Serv Res. 2014 Jan 6;14:6.

[58] Menotti A, Lanti M, Puddu PE, Carratelli L, Mancini M, Motolese M, et al. An Italian chart for cardiovascular risk prediction. Its scientific basis. Ann Ital Med Interna Organo Uff Della Soc Ital Med Int. 2001;16(4):240–51.

[59] Italian Cardiovascular Risk Estimation Research Team. Italian Cardiovascular Risk Chart. Roma: Cardioricerca, 2001.

[60] Menotti A, Lanti M, Puddu PE, Carratelli L, Mancini M, Motolese M, et al. The risk functions incorporated in Riskard 2002: a software for the prediction of cardiovascular risk in the general population based on Italian data. Ital Heart J Off J Ital Fed Cardiol. 2002;3(2):114–21.

[61] Menotti A, Lanti M, Agabiti-Rosei E, Carratelli L, Cavera G, Dormi A, et al. Riskard 2005. New tools for prediction of cardiovascular disease risk derived from Italian population studies. Nutr Metab Cardiovasc Dis NMCD. 2005;15(6):426–40.

[62] Echouffo-Tcheugui J-B, Kengne AP. Comparative performance of diabetes-specific and general population-based cardiovascular risk assessment models in people with diabetes mellitus. Diabetes Metab. 2013;39(5):389–96.

[63] Pellegrini E, Maurantonio M, Giannico IM, Simonini MS, Ganazzi D, Carulli L, et al. Risk for cardiovascular events in an Italian population of patients with type 2 diabetes. Nutr Metab Cardiovasc Dis NMCD. 2011;21(11):885–92.

[64] De Berardis G, Pellegrini F, Franciosi M, Belfiglio M, Di Nardo B, Greenfield S, et al. Quality of diabetes care predicts the development of cardiovascular events: results of the QuED study. Nutr Metab Cardiovasc Dis NMCD. 2008;18(1):57–65.

[65] Fleming BB, Greenfield S, Engelgau MM, Pogach LM, Clauser SB, Parrott MA. The Diabetes Quality Improvement Project: moving science into health policy to gain an edge on the diabetes epidemic. Diabetes Care 2001;24(10):1815–20.

[66] Heart Outcomes Prevention Evaluation (HOPE) Study Investigators. Effects of ramipril on cardiovascular and microvascular outcomes in people with diabetes mellitus: results of the HOPE study and MICRO-HOPE substudy. Heart Outcomes Prevention Evaluation Study Investigators. Lancet 2000;355(9200):253–9.

[67] Rossi MCE, Lucisano G, Comaschi M, Coscelli C, Cucinotta D, Di Blasi P, et al. Quality of diabetes care predicts the development of cardiovascular events: results of the AMD-QUASAR study. Diabetes Care 2011;34(2):347–52.

[68] Annali AMD. Annali 2010-2011-2012. Available from www.infodiabetes.it [Accessed April 22, 2015].

[69] Rossi MC, Candido R, Ceriello A, Cimino A, Di Bartolo P, Giorda C, et al. Trends over 8 years in quality of diabetes care: results of the AMD Annals continuous quality improvement initiative. Acta Diabetol. 2015;52(3):557-71.

[70] Welschen LMC, Bot SDM, Kostense PJ, Dekker JM, Timmermans DRM, van der Weijden T, et al. Effects of cardiovascular disease risk communication for patients with type 2 diabetes on risk perception in a randomized controlled trial: the @RISK study. Diabetes Care 2012;35(12):2485–92.

[71] Martell-Claros N, Aranda P, González-Albarrán O, Dalfó-Baqué A, Domínguez-Sardiña M, de la Cruz JJ, et al. Perception of health and understanding of cardiovascular risk among patients with recently diagnosed diabetes and/or metabolic syndrome. Eur J Prev Cardiol. 2013;20(1):21–8.

[72] Gianinazzi F, Bodenmann P, Izzo F, Voeffray Favre AC, Rossi I, Ruiz J. Risk perception and communication: from diabetes to cardiovascular diseases. Rev Médicale Suisse. 2010;6(252):1182–4, 1186–7.

[73] Bisconcin M, Garelli L Cardiovascular risk perception in people with diabetes: PRICAD study (Percezione del rischio cardiovascolare nel diabetico: lo studio PRICAD). M.D. Medicinae Doctor – Anno XV 2008;10:20-27.

[74] Katz M, Laurinavicius AG, Franco FG, Conceicao RD, Carvalho JA, Pesaro AE, et al. Calculated and perceived cardiovascular risk in asymptomatic subjects submitted to a routine medical evaluation: the perception gap. Eur J Prev Cardiol. 2015;22(8):1076-82.

[75] Wells S, Kerr A, Broadbent E, MacKenzie C, Cole K, McLachlan A. Does your heart forecast help practitioner understanding and confidence with cardiovascular disease risk communication? J Prim Health Care 2011;3(1):4–9.

[76] Jackson R. Cardiovascular risk prediction: are we there yet? Heart Br Card Soc. 2008;94(1):1–3.

[77] Edwards A, Elwyn G, Mulley A. Explaining risks: turning numerical data into meaningful pictures. BMJ 2002;324(7341):827–30.

[78] Wolpert HA, Anderson BJ. Management of diabetes: are doctors framing the benefits from the wrong perspective? BMJ 2001;323(7319):994–6.

Section 3

Integrated Approach in Primary Care Practice

Chapter 6

Integrated Activities in Primary Care – Minor Surgery in Family Medicine

José María Arribas Blanco, Shabnan Habibi, Nuria Rodríguez Pata and José Ramón Castello Fortet

Additional information is available at the end of the chapter

http://dx.doi.org/10.5772/62650

Abstract

Minor surgery is defined as the overall surgical procedures of short duration that are generally applied on surface structures. They usually require the application of local anaesthesia and involve performing low and minimal complication risk.

In Primary Care, often some problems need surgery techniques for diagnosis or treatment. Therefore, minor surgery must be within the field of knowledge and skills of a good family physician as a cost-effective tool more for a quality professional practice, attention both scheduled (excision of skin lesions), as in the emergency (suturing wounds).

The limiting factor for excellence in minor surgery is the technical training that makes Family Doctor. Moreover, the minor surgery is not without risks, both during the procedure and after. Therefore, it is imperative in addition to proper surgical technique and suitable directions, to offer a clear and complete information to patients, which will be reflected in the informed consent form. In addition, it is advisable to have a medical insurance with specific coverage for these techniques.

In this chapter, we intend to give scientific answers as to how?, with what ? and where? to perform minor surgery in the field of quality of primary care.

Keywords: Minor surgery, surgical procedures, fusiform excision, suturing techniques, primary care

1. Introduction

Minor surgery (MS) is defined as the group of surgical techniques of a short duration that are generally applied to superficial structures. They tend to require the application of local anaesthesia and involve little risk and a minimum degree of complications [1].

INTECH
open science | open minds

© 2016 The Author(s). Licensee InTech. This chapter is distributed under the terms of the Creative Commons Attribution License (http://creativecommons.org/licenses/by/3.0), which permits unrestricted use, distribution, and reproduction in any medium, provided the original work is properly cited.

During Primary Care consultations, one frequently comes across health problems that require these procedures for treatment and diagnosis. For this reason, MS falls within the fields of knowledge and competences [2] of a Family Physician (FP), being an additional cost-effective tool [3–5] for quality professional practices [6], both during programmed clinical treatments (excision of skin disorders) and in case of emergency (stitching of injuries).

The fundamental component for excellent MS is the technical capability of the FP carrying it out [1, 4, 7]. On the other hand, MS is not exempt from risk, either while it is being carried out or afterwards. It is therefore essential that, in addition to carrying out correct technical surgical procedures [8, 9] as appropriately indicated [10, 11], we also offer the patient a clear and complete information, which will be set out in the informed consent form. Furthermore, it is highly recommended that there should be some form of insurance available with specific cover for such techniques [12].

In this section, our aim is to provide scientific responses as to where? with what? and how? quality MS should be carried out by the FP.

2. Recommended infrastructure for a minor surgery room

In order to carry out MS, there are some basic requirements with regard to infrastructure and furnishings [1, 13].

2.1. The room

The recommended size is in the order of 15–20 m^2, with adequate temperature, well ventilated and a good source of artificial light. The ideal situation is to have a room set aside exclusively for MS procedures (Figure 1), although it is sufficient to have a well-prepared treatment room. It is very recommendable that the room should have a wash basin with a single-action tap control and an automatic soap dispenser for washing hands.

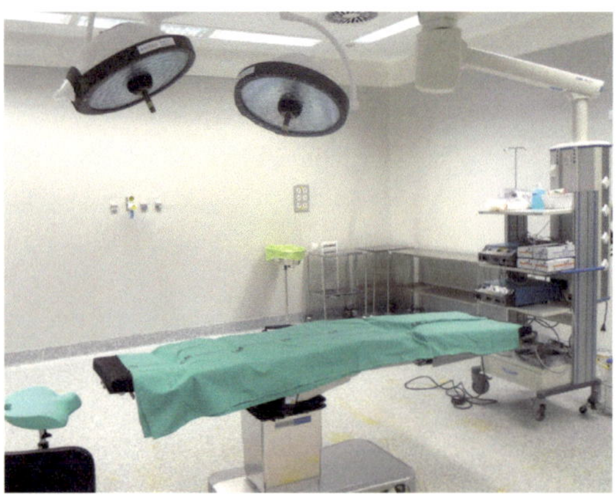

Figure 1. Well equipped minor surgery room

http://dx.doi.org/10.5772/62650

2.2. Stretcher

This should be located in the centre of the room so that it can be accessed from all sides. It is recommended that it should be height-adjustable so that the operator can work comfortably, whether seated or standing. Clinical examination benches are not acceptable.

2.3. Auxiliary table

An auxillary table is for setting out the materials and instruments used during the surgical procedure. It should have wheels and be height-adjustable and should be placed close to the area of the surgical procedure in order to facilitate the treatment. We should avoid placing any surgical materials on top of the patient.

2.4. Stool for the doctor

There should be a stool available for the doctor's use, which should have wheels and be height-adjustable so that the MS can be carried out comfortably.

2.5. Lamp

This should provide the appropriate amount of light, having an illumination level of at least 45,000 lux. It can be portable with wheels or be attached to a wall or to the ceiling. These lamps can be moved in various directions. The intensity of the luminosity can be modified, and the focal point of the light can be concentrated. It is recommended that there should also be an auxiliary lamp with a magnifying glass, which is useful for extracting foreign bodies or for working with magnification.

2.6. Resuscitation equipment

Although risks to life are minimal during MS, it is essential that there should be a carriage available with cardiopulmonary resuscitation equipment on it, carrying the materials for vascular access, intubation of the air passages, serums, resuscitation medication and a defibrillator.

2.7. Sterilisation system

The centre in which MS procedures are carried out should have an autoclave for sterilising surgical materials and equipment, or an external circuit should be set up so that the material can be sterilised.

2.8. Glass cabinet and containers

These are useful for the storage of perishable materials and surgical instruments. Likewise, there should be containers available for biocontaminated materials and an elimination system that conforms to the sanitary legislation in force at the time.

3. The FP's preparation for minor surgery

In the area of primary care, where teamwork is a key to the realization of all clinical activities, the work of the nurse is also a key for successful accomplishment of minor surgery techniques. In many cases, it is the perfect surgical assistant for preoperative, operative and postoperative and in other cases as lead actor of surgery, suturing wounds or performing cryosurgery techniques. In either case, the good cooperation between doctor and nurse entails highly efficient outcomes for the patients.

Furthermore, carrying out MS involves the risk of transmission of infectious and contagious diseases. Universal precautionary steps should be taken in order to minimise this risk. Among these steps are the use of appropriate clothing and accessories and the correct washing of hands and the sterile donning of surgical gloves [1, 14].

3.1. Clothing

During MS procedures, we consider the wearing of an overall to be essential (disposable overalls are very useful) or at least sterile pyjamas and gloves; highly recommended are the use of a surgical mask and of protective glasses or goggles.

3.2. Washing of hands

There are different methods; thus, we have *hygienic washing,* lasting a minimum of 20 seconds, which is carried out using a soapy or antiseptic hand-washing solution (no brush) correctly rubbing all of the folds of the hands. This method of washing is appropriate for MS, whereas anatomic washing (which lasts longer and is more laborious) is more appropriate for major surgery. It is important that no more than 10 minutes should elapse between the washing of the hands and the donning of sterile gloves.

3.3. Donning of gloves

Surgical gloves are sterile, single use and are available in several sizes (numbered [from 6½ to 8½] or alpha-numeric [XS, S, M, L and XL]. There are models with or without latex and with or without a dusted coating.

Surgical gloves are put on in such a way as to avoid them becoming contaminated. The dusted or internal part of the glove can be touched with the hands, whereas the external or non-dusted part should only be touched with the other glove.

4. Necessary materials

4.1. Instruments for minor surgery

The FP should have in-depth knowledge of the surgical instruments and their use. The quality and the type of instrument (and its state of conservation) can affect the result of the surgical

http://dx.doi.org/10.5772/62650

technique; that is, why it is important to correctly select the appropriate instrument for each intervention [1, 13]. The most significant characteristics of the instruments recommended for minor surgery are described below.

4.1.1. Scalpel

This enables sharp cuts to be made to the skin and other tissues and precise dissections of tissue to be carried out. It should have a number 3 handle and number 15 and 11 blades. The scalpel blade should be attached to the handle in a single position, making the guide of the blade coincides with that of the handle.

It is handled with the dominant hand, even though it was a pencil (Figure 2), enabling small and precise incisions to be made. The hand should be partially supported by the work surface in order to ensure the precision of the cut. The opposing hand should be used to stretch the skin in a direction that is perpendicular to that of the incision. The scalpel should make a cut that is perpendicular to the skin (not bevelled), except in hairy areas (the scalp or eyebrows) where it should be inclined so that it is parallel to the direction in which the hair comes out, so as not to affect the follicles.

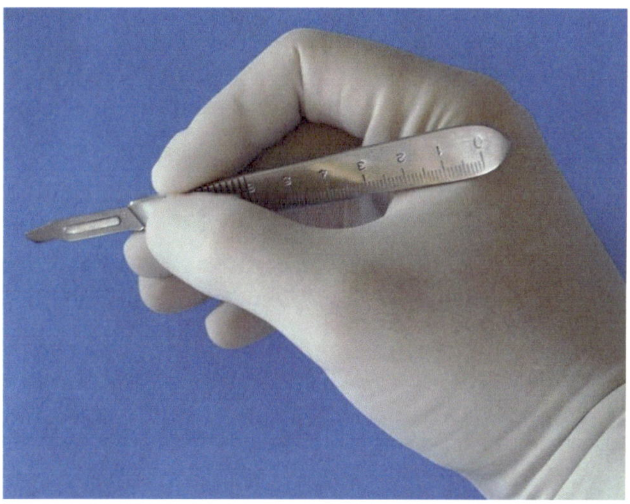

Figure 2. The knife is held with the dominant hand, as if it were a pencil

4.1.2. Needle holder

The needle holders, or "holders", are designed to safely hold the curved needles without damaging them (the points or grips are appropriate for holding the needles). The needle is held somewhere between the middle and the back third of said needle. It is recommended that there should be standard small- or medium-sized holders (12–15 cm.) with tips capable of handling needles of up to 4/0.

Like other instruments with finger rings, the needle holder is handled by partially introducing the distal phalanges of the thumb and the index finger of the dominant hand, with the index finger pointing towards the tip (Figure 3). When carrying out a stitch, the holder should describe a pronation–supination movement to facilitate the passage of the needle through the tissue. The angle of entry of the needle through the skin should be 90° while the non-dominant hand holds the skin with dissecting forceps, in opposition to the pressure of the needle.

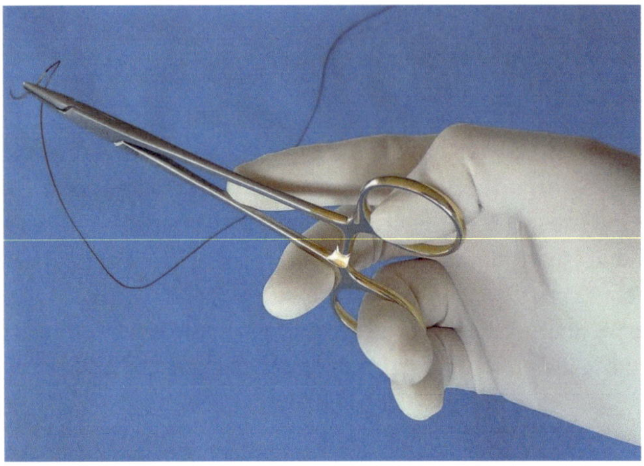

Figure 3. The needle- holders is managed partly by introducing the distal phalanges of the thumb and fourth finger of the dominant hand on the rings, while the index is directed towards the tip.

4.1.3. Dissecting forceps

There should be some toothed Adson forceps, 12 cm in length, for handling the skin, and some untoothed Adson forceps for the removal of stitches. Otherwise, standard small forceps should be used. It is important not to handle the skin with untoothed forceps.

Dissecting forceps are the most important of the auxiliary instruments used with the non-dominant hand; they enable the tissues that are handled, dissected or stitched to be exposed while the other hand uses the main instrument. The forceps are held like a pencil between the first, second and third fingers.

4.1.4. Scissors

These enable the cutting of both cloth and materials (sutures, bandages and dressings), as well as the dissection of tissues. There should be curved Mayo (cutting) scissors with blunt tips, 14 cm in length, and curved Metzembaum (dissecting) scissors with blunt tips, 11.5 cm in length. The dissecting scissors are not recommended for cutting materials. They are handled by introducing part of the distal phalanges of the thumb and fourth finger into the finger rings, supporting the second finger on the arms of the instrument.

For blunt dissection, the Metzembaum scissors are introduced with the tips closed, and these are then opened separating the tissues through more or less anatomical layers. For cutting

http://dx.doi.org/10.5772/62650

dissections, the scissors are introduced with the tips open, and these are then closed cutting the tissue.

4.1.5. Haemostatic forceps

There should be two or three sets of curved 12-cm untoothed mosquito forceps. These should be used for creating traction in tissues for haemostasis and in some cases for carrying out blunt dissection when we have no scissors available.

4.1.6. Surgical retractors

These enable the surgical field to be exposed by separating or retracting the edges of the injury. If the surgery is being carried out with the help of an assistant, it will be he or she who uses the retractors; otherwise, it will be the surgeon who uses them with the non-dominant hand. In MS, it is recommendable to have a Senn-Mueller retractor (with a scoop on one end and curved tynes on the other). Another useful retractor in MS is a hook or distractor.

4.1.7. Additional expendable materials

Additional expendable materials are single-use gauze dressings, sterile dressings and bandages, antiseptics (iodised povidone [polyvinylpyrrolidone]), needles, syringes, local anaesthetics with and without vasoconstrictors (see local anaesthetic guide) and formaldehyde for transfers to anatomic pathology.

To perform the majority of MS techniques, only a **basic instrument set** is needed (Figure 4). However, certain Primary Care surgical procedures require special instrumentation or equipment, such as curettes, punches, electrical scalpels, cryosurgery materials and surgical retractors.

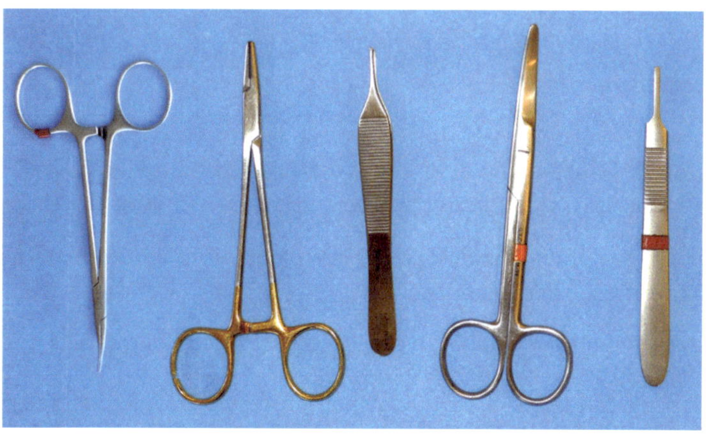

Figure 4. Starter Kit minor surgery. From left to right, curved mosquito forceps without teeth, needle holders medium Asson dissecting forceps, scissors Mayo, Scalpel Handle number 3

4.1.8. Curettes

Instruments consisting of a handle with an end in the shape of a small spoon or cutting ring enable the scraping of injuries on the surface of the skin. They can be disposable or not and have different diameters. The curette is handled with the dominant hand in accordance with the surgical technique known as "scraping" or enucleating benign superficial skin lesions (protruding or hyperkerastotic) that do not require histological confirmation [15].

4.1.9. Biopsy punches

Instruments consisting of a handle with an end in the shape of a cutting cylinder (drill bit) enable tissue biopsies to be extracted. They tend to be disposable and can have different diameters (from 2 to 28 mm.) and enable samples to be taken of the full thickness of the useful skin for histological analysis. They are used with the dominant hand carrying out rotating movements of the instrument in order to cut the skin and obtain the sample [16].

4.1.10. Cryosurgical equipment

These devices apply a cryogen, generally liquid nitrogen, by means of pulverization or swabs to treat skin lesions [17]. The cryogen is stored in tanks or containers in order to avoid its evaporation. There are portable units available which have a mechanism for pulverising the nitrogen over the lesion to be treated; they are equipped with a range of outlets and probes, which enable the intensity of the pulverisation to be modified, thus varying the amount applied depending on the size and location of the lesion to be treated.

4.1.11. Electrical scalpel

Electrical apparatus consists of a central unit that applies an electrical current through a sterile terminal, with the capacity to coagulate and cut; it also consists of an earth to close the electrical circuit [18]. There are different terminals available depending on the type of procedure to be carried out.

4.2. Care of instruments

With appropriate care, surgical instruments last a long time. The majority of the damage that they suffer is due to incorrect cleaning and handling. On the other hand, MS instruments should always be used in a sterile state. The steps taken care of these details are as follows:

1. Separate sharp or pointed single-use objects (using gloves) and dispose of them in the biocontaminated materials container.

2. The instruments should be placed in disinfecting solutions (a glutaraldehyde or clorhexidine solution at 0.05%, etc.) or a soapy solution.

3. Sterilising. The most appropriate and recommended method is to use an autoclave to control the quality of the sterilisation process.

4. Packaging and labelling.

http://dx.doi.org/10.5772/62650

4.3. Suturing materials

There are different types of materials available: threads, staples, adhesive sutures and tissue adhesives. The use of a certain type of suturing material or type of needle can determine differences in the surgical result, so the choice should be based on scientific criteria and be backed up by good practice.

Thread sutures provide a sure close and ensure the greatest support for the wound and the minimum level of dehiscence compared to other types of closure [19, 20]; however, they require anaesthesia, the intervention takes longer, they traumatise the tissue, introduce foreign bodies into the wound and increase the risk of accidental inoculation.

The alternatives to conventional sutures are mechanical sutures and adhesive tapes, which provide less reactivity and a lower degree of incidence of infections [21]. Glues and tissue adhesives have appeared as an option to common procedures [22–25].

4.3.1. Suture threads

These are classified in accordance with: their origin (natural or synthetic), their configuration (multifilament or monofilament), their calibre (the thickness of the thread is measured in zeros [USP system] with the fewer zeros meaning lower calibre and the most commonly used in minor surgery ranging from 3/0 to 4/0 or 5/0, the finer calibres with smaller needles requiring more precise needle holders) (Figure 5).

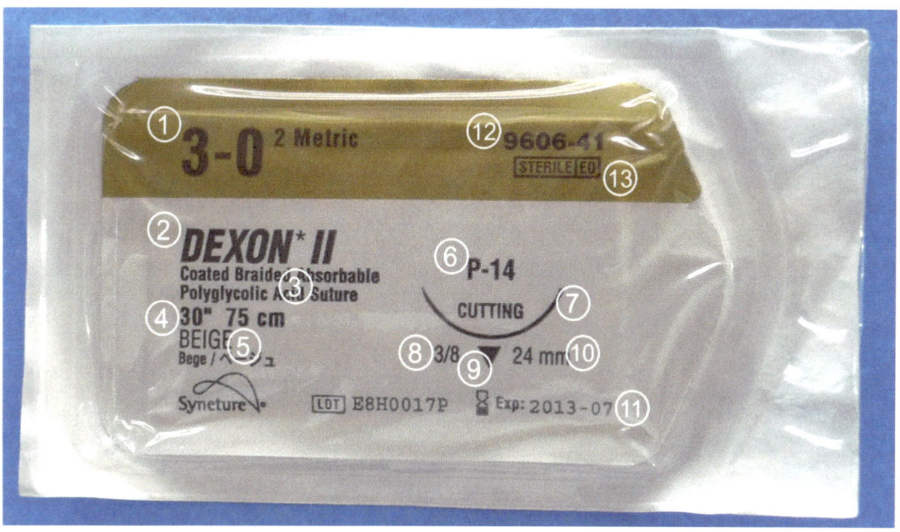

Figure 5. Information of on of suture: (1) calibre of the thread (system USP and metric), (2) trade name of the suture, (3) composition and physical structure of the thread, (4) length of the thread, (5) color of the thread, (6) model of needle (every manufacturer uses different references), (7) I draw from the needle to scale 1:1, (8) circumference of the needle (expressed in parts of circle), (9) section of the needle, (10) length of the needle, (11) expiry date, (12) indexes of the manufacturer, (13) indicator of sterile packing.

We will use a certain type and thickness of suture thread depending on the anatomical area and the characteristics of the wound and the patient (Table 1).

Anatomical region	**Skin suturing**	**Subcutaneous suturing (whenever necessary)**	**Stitch removal**	
			Adults	**children**
Scalp	staples 2/0 silk	Vicryl® or Dexon® 3/0	7–9	6–8
Eyelids	6/0 monofilament 6/0 silk	-	3–5	3–5
Ears	4/0-5/0 monofilament 4/0-5/0 silk	-	4–5	3–5
Nose	4/0 monofilament 4/0 silk	Vicryl® or Dexon® 4/0	4–6	3–5
Lips	4/0 monofilament 4/0 silk	Vicryl® or Dexon® 4/0	4–6	4–5
Forehead and face Neck	4/0–5/0 monofilament 4/0–5/0 silk	Vicryl® or Dexon® 4/0	4–6	3–5
Trunk / abdomen	3/0–4/0 monofilament	Vicryil® or Dexon® 3/0	7–12	7–9
Back	3/0–4/0 monofilament	Vicryil® or Dexon® 3/0	12–14	14
Upper limb / hand	4/0 monofilament	Vicryil® or Dexon® 3/0	8–10	7–9
Pulp of fingers	4/0 monofilament	-	10–12	8–10
Lower extremity	3/0 monofilamentstaples	Vicryil® or Dexon® 3/0	8–12	7–10
Foot	4/0 monofilament	Vicryil® or Dexon® 3/0	10–12	8–10
Penis	4/0 monofilament	Vicryil® or Dexon® 3/0	7–10	6–8
Mouth and tongue	3/0 Vicryil®	-	-	-

Table 1. Indications of types of sutures and time for stitch removal

4.3.1.1. Characteristics of the suture threads

Non-absorbable sutures

These are used for skin sutures that will be removed or for internal structures that need to maintain constant pressure (tendons and ligaments).

1. Silk: Indicated for skin suturing and generally extractable, however, they do cause significant tissue reaction.

2. Nylon: Indicated for precise skin suturing, internal structures that need to maintain constant pressure (tendons and nerves). They are more difficult to handle but produce minimum tissue reaction.

http://dx.doi.org/10.5772/62650

3. Polypropylene: Indicated for continuous intradermal skin sutures. They are very smooth sutures with a long memory, so they require more knotting so that they do not come undone. They cause minimum tissue reaction.

Absorbable sutures

These disappear gradually by biological reabsorption or hydrolysis and provoke localised inflammation. They are used for deep or non-extractable suturing.

1. Polyglactin 910: Indicated for dermal sutures, subcutaneous cellular tissue, deep suturing and the ligature of small vessels. They have an absorption time of 60 days (conserving tissue support for 28–30 days). There are varieties with a quicker absorption time (Vicryl®rapid) that are absorbed in 10 days and are used for the suturing of children's skin.
2. Polyglycolic acid: Indications similar to the above. They have an absorption time of 90 days and the support of 15–20 days.

4.3.1.2. Removal of stitches

The time (in days) recommended for the removal of stitches together with the indication of the type of suture thread is shown in Table 1.

In the face, it is important to remove the sutures as soon as possible, although adhesive sutures are put in place for an additional 7 days to protect the wound against small traumatisms. In other anatomical regions where the aesthetic result is not as important and scarring is not as quick as in the face, stitches should be left in for longer. In particular, in periarticular regions and in the lower extremities, which have a slower scarring time, stitches are left in for longer than normal.

4.3.2. Suture needles

The needles are designed to take the suture through the tissue producing minimum damage. The selection of these is determined by the type of tissue to be sutured, its accessibility and the thickness of the thread used. There are *straight needles* that are handled using the fingers, which are not used in MS, and *curved needles* that are handled using a needle holder, enabling greater precision; these have different circumference arcs, with those describing 3/8 of a circle or 1/2 of a circle being the most widely used in MS.

The section of the needle can be triangular, conical or spatula-shaped. The triangular ones have cutting edges that enable them to pass through highly resistant tissue, such as skin and subcutaneous tissue, these being the needle of choice for MS.

4.3.3. Adhesive sutures

The adhesive sutures consist of porous adhesive paper tape (Steri-Strip®, etc.) capable of bringing the edges of a wound or incision together. They are available in sterile presentations with different widths and lengths although they can be cut to the appropriate size as required. Advantage of adhesive sutures is the speed and simplicity of application when compared to conventional sutures because they do not require local anaesthesia and they do not leave "stitch marks".

Indications: For linear and superficial wounds that little tension there, as in the forehead, chin, the malar eminence, the thorax and the pads of the fingers. They are also a good choice for the elderly (or in treatments with corticoids) where the skin is fine and fragile and for reinforcing wounds after the removal of stitches.

Contraindications: Their use on irregular wounds where there is pressure or on wounds where bleeding or secretions cannot be stopped. They are not indicated for use on the scalp or hairy areas, folds in the skin and jointed surfaces.

Application and removal of adhesive sutures: The wound should be dry, free of blood or secretions; substances can be added to increase the adhesiveness of the skin. The adhesive suture is cut, before the removal of paper, to the required size and is then applied using untoothed dissecting forceps or the fingers, first along one edge of the wound and then the other and along the length of the wound.

Adhesive sutures are left for as long as a conventional suture would be left in the same anatomical region. Unlike other sutures, a wound with adhesive sutures should not be allowed to get wet during the first few days because of the possibility that they will become unstuck.

4.3.4. Staples

Staples are available in different widths (W: wide staples, R: normal staples), in disposable staplers preloaded with a varying number of staples (35 in the case of large staplers and 10 for smaller ones). The use of staples as compared to conventional sutures has certain advantages, such as the speed with which the suturing is carried out, their resistance and null tissue reaction (the material is stainless steel).

Indications (1): In linear injuries to the scalp, the trunk and the extremities and, for the temporary closure of wounds, in patients who are going to be transferred to another specialised service.

Contraindications: On the face and hands. In areas where a TAC or MRN scan is to be carried out.

Application and removal of staples: The staples are applied with the dominant hand, whereas the non-dominant hand brings the edges of the skin closer and everts or overturns them. Staples are kept in place for the same length of time as a conventional suture would be kept in the same anatomical region. The removal of the staples is carried out using a staple remover.

4.3.5. Tissue adhesives (glues)

One of the latest advances in the treatment of wounds has been the development of tissue adhesives or tissue glues (22, 23). These products (cyanoacrylates) act as an adhesive, using an effect of joining the epidermal layer (the stratum corneatum), thus keeping the edges of the wound joined together. The compound forms a bridge over the edges of the wound creating

http://dx.doi.org/10.5772/62650

an effective joint during a period of 7–14 days. After this time, the major part of the compound is loosened and detached, together with the *stratum corneatum,* before degradation takes place.

Application technique: After placing the patient in a *decubitus* position and cleaning the wound well and stemming the blood flow, the following steps are taken:

- Bring the edges of the wound together precisely using the fingers or dissecting forceps.
- Apply the glue to the external surface of the skin, avoiding it penetrating inside the wound. The application process is repeated at least three or four times.
- Keep the edges in contact for 30–60 seconds to achieve an adequate degree of polymerization. The final tension is produced 2 minutes after application.
- After application, no dressings are required. The wound should be kept dry for 5 days and subsequently it can be moistened with care, avoiding prolonged contact with water. The glue will disappear after a period of 7–10 days.

Indications: Tissue adhesives are a good alternative for the closure of wounds that meet the following criteria [1, 22]:

- They would require 4/0 sutures or finer.
- They are not associated with multiple trauma.
- The patients do not have any peripheral vascular illness, diabetes mellitus, haemorrhagic diathesis or a history of the formation of keloids.
- The cause is not an animal bite, puncturing, decubitus ulcers or injuries arising from crushing, which provokes star-shaped lesions.
- There are no visual signs of active local or systematic infection, visible contamination or lifeless tissue.
- They are not localised around the pigmented edges of the lips in the mucous areas or in areas covered in dense hair.

5. Basic surgical manoeuvres

The practicing of MS requires a knowledge of the correct handling of surgical instruments (described above) and control of the consecutive steps of each surgical technique: that is to say, capabilities in surgical manoeuvres.

5.1. Surgical incision and dissection

Dissection is a manoeuvre that consists of detaching layers of similar tissue. There are two methods for carrying it out: one is called blunt dissection (non-cutting which is generally carried out with Metzembaun scissors or with mosquito forceps) and the other known as cutting, where a scalpel or scissors are used. In MS, the more frequent degree of dissection should be for the face and neck, which corresponding to the joint between the dermis and the subcutaneous tissue, and for the scalp, the subgalea layer and for the trunk and the extremities, which corresponding to the joint between the superficial and the profound fascias [26).

Dissection manoeuvres must be carried out in a delicate manner and with the field of operation well exposed, never obscured, so as not to damage important structures in an irreversible manner; it is therefore fundamental that one knows the topographic anatomy of the area being operated.

5.1.1. Incisions in MS

The design of the incisions should be done bearing in mind that the type of lesion that is to be treated so, for excisions, it is necessary to leave an adequate margin (1–2 mm) of healthy skin around the wound and in depth, depending on each wound. On many occasions, it is useful to mark out the planned excision so that reference points are not lost when surgical swabs are put in place.

Likewise, when planning a surgical incision, it is necessary to take into account the anatomy of the area to be operated upon and the lines of minimum tension; in this way, an appropriate scar will result both from an aesthetic and from a functional point of view. It is therefore necessary to direct incisions parallel to the lines of minimum tension (coinciding with the lines of facial expression and the lines of cutaneous relaxation; Figure 6).

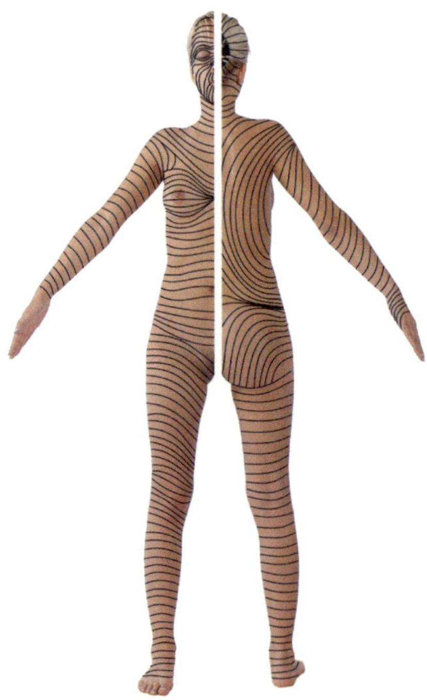

Figure 6. Graphs of the lines of minimal tension (the lines of Langers)

http://dx.doi.org/10.5772/62650

5.1.2. Types of incisions in MS

5.1.2.1. Incision

These are used to achieve a surgical exposure of the more profound layers (e.g., epidermal cysts, lipomas) or for the draining of ulcers. They can be lineal, angled, or curved depending on the anatomical area to be treated and the type of surgery.

5.1.2.2. Fusiform excisions

These are used to extract cutaneous lesions with a margin of healthy skin around the wound and in depth [27, 28]. As a general rule, the length of the ellipse should be three times its width and the ends should have angles of 30° (Figure 7). They should be directed in accordance with the lines of minimum tension not according to the major axis of the wound.

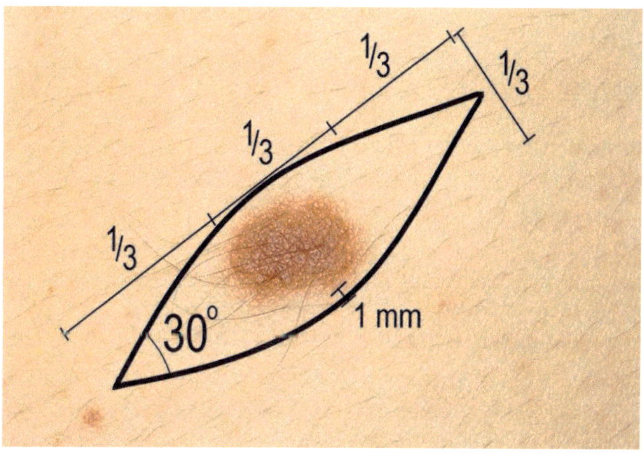

Figure 7. Characteristics of the fusiform excision.

5.1.2.3. Tangential excision

These are also known as "shaved" and consist of the extraction with a scalpel or scissors of very superficial lesions, which would scar at a second attempt. They should only be carried out on certain lesions which leave no element of diagnostic doubt [28, 29].

5.2. Haemostasis

This is a surgical manoeuvre that enables not only the control of bleeding but also a clarifying of the view of the surgical anatomy. The majority of haemorrhages in MS (where incisions or wounds do not tend to affect important vessels) are controllable with pressure using a gauze. On the other hand, a compress bandage over the wound during the immediate post-operative period reduces the possibility of bruising or seromas forming.

5.2.1. *Types of haemostasis*

- The *torniquet* is not a method of haemostasis "per se", although it does provide a temporary control of the haemorrhage enabling the wound to be explored and reducing the time of surgery. Its use in MS is limited to the fingers (surgery of nails, etc.) and should not exceed 15 minutes.
- *Haemostasis forceps.* After identifying the vessel that is bleeding, it is pinched using the tips of untoothed haemostasis forceps, ensuring that when they are clamped the haemorrhage ceases. Attempts at blind clamping a bleeding vessel in the depths of a wound should be avoided because of the risk of damaging important structures.
- *Ligatures* are threads that are tied around a blood vessel to occlude light and avoid the haemorrhage. After identifying the bleeding vessel, it is held by means of haemostasis forceps and a thread (absorbable 3/0 thread) is passed below the forceps and tied. The ends are left short.
- Haemostasis by means of *electrocoagulation* uses an electrical scalpel as a means of coagulation.

5.3. Suturing techniques

The objective of a suture is to draw tissues with similar characteristics together so that they can scar correctly. To achieve an optimum surgical closure, the principles shown in Table 2 should be taken into account [30, 31].

1. **Tension must be avoided**: Suturing a wound under tension decreases the blood supply to its edges, increasing healing problems and the risk of infection.
2. **Eversion of the wound edges**: Due to the tendency of scars to contract over time, if surgical edges are left slightly elevated above the plane of the skin, they will flatten over time, producing a more cosmetically acceptable result. One of the keys to proper surgical skin edge eversion is to introduce the needle at a 90° angle with the plane of the skin so that the suture, once tied, lifts the skin
3. **Closure by layers**: For most minor surgical interventions, a single (cutaneous) layer closure is enough. However, if there is any tension, if the wound is very deep and involves several surgical layers or if there is much dead space, a multilayer closure may become necessary. A multilayer wound closure requires thick fascia or dermis for the placement of internal sutures because fatty tissue lacks consistency to support sutures.
4. **Type of suture material**: It is a less important factor than the previous principles. If a suture is removed too late, it will cause scarring in the areas of entry and exit of the suture ("cross-hatching"). To avoid it, stitches shall be removed as soon points as possible. The choice of suture material and its thickness are also important.

Table 2. For an optimal surgical closure, the following principles should be remembered

5.3.1. *Discontinuous sutures*

Discontinuous sutures are those where each stitch is independent of the following one. They are the most appropriate for MS because it is easier to distribute the tension, favouring the drainage of the wound. Also, the stitches can be removed more easily.

http://dx.doi.org/10.5772/62650

5.3.1.1. Simple stitch (percutaneous)

This is the suture of choice for suturing skin and is only used in combination with buried stitches if the wound is deeper.

5.3.1.2. Simple stitch with an inverted knot (buried)

This is used for drawing together the deeper layers, reducing the tension and for obliterating empty spaces before suturing of the skin; it is not necessary for superficial wounds. Absorbable materials are used, and the suturing is carried out in such a way that the knot is left in the depths of the wound, reducing the possibility that the stitch might be exposed through the incision. The knot is cut right down to reduce the amount of foreign matter inside the wound.

5.3.1.3. "U" or 'Upholsterer's stitch'

This is a double stitch that increases the resistance of the suture but is more aggressive around the edges of the wound. There are three types [30, 32]:

1. *Vertical*: Apart from producing good eversion or overturning of the edges of the wound, it adequately obliterates empty spaces at depth. It is useful in areas of flaccid skin (the backs of hands and elbows), where the scar tends to invaginate or fold inwardly.
2. *Horizontal*: This suture also provides good eversion of the edges of the wound, above all in areas where the dermis is thick (palm of the hand or sole of the foot).
3. *Horizontal semi-buried Upholsterer's stitch*: This is used to suture corners of wounds or surgical edges with different thicknesses.

5.3.2. Continuous sutures

These make the drainage of the wound more difficult, so they are contraindicated if there is a suspicion of infection or in very contaminated wounds. The stitches are more difficult to remove, and it is not possible to remove them in various sessions [30].

5.3.2.1. Simple continuous suture

This is a succession of stitches with an initial knot and another at the other end. It is scarcely used in MS.

5.3.2.2. Continuous intradermal sutures (subcuticular)

This type of suture enables the suturing to be carried out without passing through the skin, avoiding scarring from "stitch marks" and providing an optimum aesthetic result. They are carried out by passing the suture through the dermis in a horizontal manner, along the length of the whole wound; at the ends, the suture can appear outside the skin (extractable intradermal suture), in which case it is carried out with non-absorbable monofilament material, or it can be knotted inside the wound (non-extractable intradermal suture), in which case absorbable material is used. Carrying out this suture with multifilament materials, such as silk, should be avoided, as it would be very difficult to remove the suturing material. It is used in wounds where it is necessary to maintain the stitch in place for a long time (more than 15 days). Its use in MS is limited.

5.3.3. Knotted

Instrumental knotting is carried out using the needle holder and curved needles. In MS, where the surgical area is superficial and accessible to instruments, instrumental knotting is the preferred technique, as it provides greater precision in the suture, except where the ligaturing of small blood vessels is concerned where is it preferable to carry out *manual knotting* (which is carried out with the fingers).

The knot that the surgeon should use consists of a double loop followed by various simple loops. The advantage of this knot is the safety that is provided by the first double loop, which avoids the knot untying while the following loops are carried out.

If the knot is tied with a multifilament thread (silk) then three loops are sufficient; if it is monofilament (nylon, polypropylene), it is preferable to carry out a further loop.

It is convenient for the knot to be placed to one side of the wound rather than on top of the incision. This enables a better view of the wound, it interferes less with scarring and facilitates the removal of the stitches.

6. Considerations prior to minor surgery

6.1. Diagnosis of the lesion to be treated

The indications for MS are carried out on the basis of the diagnosis of the lesion to be treated; an erroneous diagnosis can lead to incorrect treatment and to the loss of clinical information that is relevant to the patient's prognosis [8]. It is therefore essential that the FP should have extensive knowledge of the lesions that are most frequently susceptible to MS and, should there be any doubts regarding the nature of the lesion, these should always be resolved through consultation with other specialists [10, 11, 33, 34]. Each lesion has a surgical procedure that is considered to be optimum or of choice, whereas other alternatives are merely valid or can be contraindicated [1, 13].

6.2. Areas of the body at risk from MS

There are certain areas of the body that are considered to be at risk when MS procedures are carried out. This is due to the superficial location of anatomic structures, susceptible to damage during the surgical intervention. To avoid damaging these structures, it is necessary to know their theoretical routing and keep the surgery, wherever possible, on a superficial level (subcutaneous superficial cellular tissue). Furthermore certain areas (face, neck) are also considered at risk by the aesthetic impact of poor technique may result [1].

http://dx.doi.org/10.5772/62650

The areas at risk during MS include the facial and cervical regions, the axillary and supraclavicular regions, the wrists, hands and fingers, the groin area, the popliteal fossa and the feet (Figure 8A and 8B).

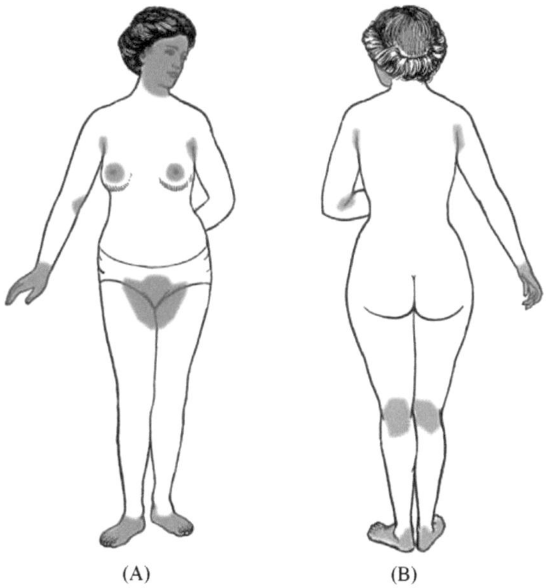

Figure 8. A and B. MS risk areas in Family Medicine

Together with the above considerations, we should also consider those anatomical areas with a greater tendency for pathological scarring: the deltoid region, shoulder, area of the sternum and the interscapular region. Also, the skin of black patients and children is especially prone to the appearance of hypertrophic scars and keloids. Therefore, in these cases, it is important to discuss these possibilities with the patients, especially if there are only aesthetic reasons for the surgery.

6.3. Histological diagnosis

All lesions extracted during MS should be sent on to a pathological anatomy service so that the correct diagnosis can be carried out. No intervention will finish without such results being available [1].

7. Procedures in MS

During MS in Primary Care, different procedures are carried out, which would each, in their own right, be the object of action protocols (the extraction of lipomas, epidermal cysts, ingrown toenails, punched biopsies, curettes, cryosurgery of benign lesions). For this reason, the main and ideal techniques for dealing with the majority of these superficial dermatological lesions through MS are summarised below.

7.1. Fusiform excision

This is an exeresis technique designed in the form of a spindle; this spindle should involve all levels of the skin, including the fatty tissues, so as to extract the lesions with a margin of safety on the surface and in the depths of the lesion. Thus, the technique enables not only a histological diagnosis and simultaneous treatment but also a closing suture that is technically simple with very good aesthetic results [27, 35].

The procedure consists of the following steps:

1. **Design of the excision,** which is marked out with a marker pen following these parameters: The longitudinal axis of the spindle will be three times greater than the transverse diameter and parallel to the lines of cutaneous tension, and the angle at the ends will be <30° so as to avoid the appearance in the scar of "dog's ears". There must be a margin between the lesion and the excision of 1–2 mm (or greater, depending upon the lesion to be extracted).

2. **Preparation of the surgical field:** cleaning and disinfection.

3. **Anaesthetic infiltration**, covering all of the edge of the incision and the tissue that is to be sectioned or sutured.

4. **Superficial cutaneous incision** along the length of the spindle, affecting all of the dermis in order to avoid irregular edges. The incision is carried out by means of a clean cut with a scalpel, not sawing, grabbing the handle of the scalpel like a pencil, tractioning (or pinching) the area with the fingers of the non-dominant hand and following the line marked out by the design (Figure 9).

5. **Block excision:** traction is carried out with the non-dominant hand (using toothed forceps) from the end of the spindle and, with the blade of the scalpel, a deep incision is made (always with a direct view in the form of a wedge until fatty tissue is reached, so that the lesion can then be extracted as a block).

6. **Haemostasis** of the surgical area: in general, if we are using anaesthesia with vasoconstriction, there is little bleeding and haemostasis is achieved using finger pressure with a gauze.

7. **Suturing** of the wound by layers: the majority of MS interventions only require the closure of the superficial cutaneous layer. However, if there is tension, if the incision is deep and involves several layers or if there is an empty area, then closure on several levels may be required. The suturing of the deepest layer should be carried out with absorbable sutures using inverted stitches. Subsequently, the superficial suturing is carried out using non-absorbable sutures. The number of stitches will depend on the tension on the wound, the thickness of the thread and the type of closure.

8. **Placing of a sterile dressing,** following the cleaning of the area.

9. **Dispatching of the extracted element to pathological anatomy,** in a container with formaldehyde at 10%.

10. **Monitoring:** After 48 hours, the wound can be washed softly and the patient should be warned of the post-surgical risks and advised about self nursing of the surgical wound. The patient will be given an appointment for the removal of the stitches and to inform him or her of the histological results.

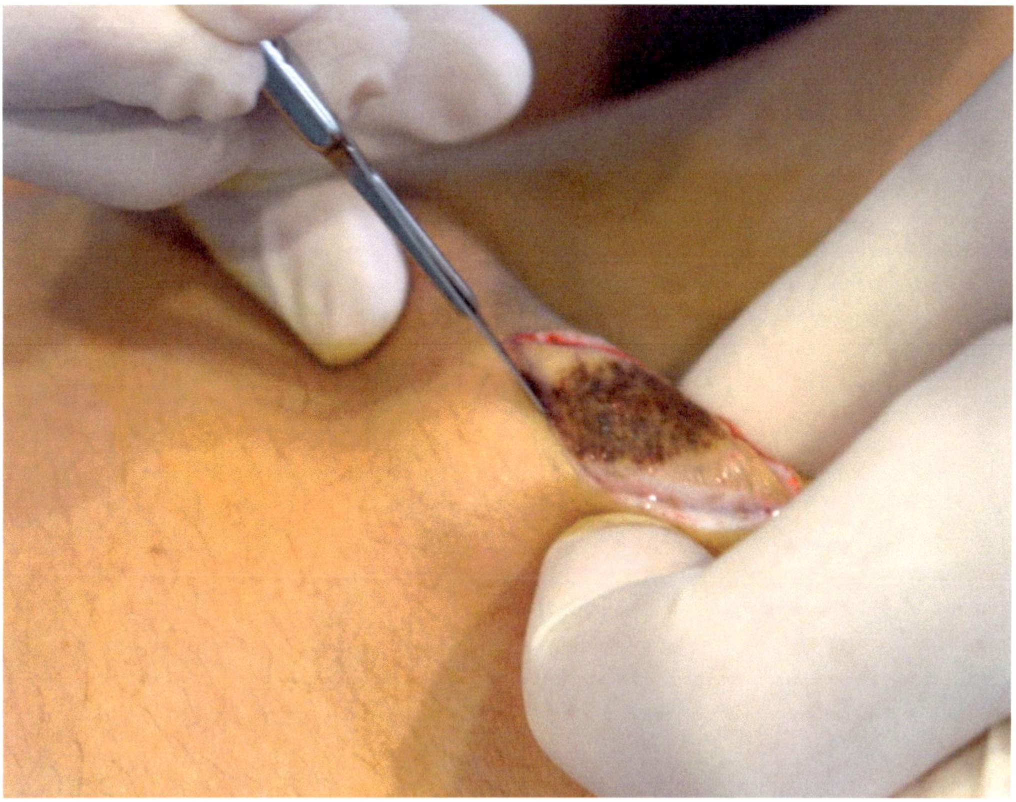

Figure 9. The incision is made with a clean knife cut along the line painted design, while we traction (or pinching the area) with the fingers of the nondominant hand

8. Good clinical practice in MS [1]

8.1. Pre-operatory study

During basic minor surgical interventions, it is not in general necessary to carry out a systematic pre-operatory study. However, as we are dealing with our own patients, we will have their medical history available, which we will complement with a series of questions directed towards evaluating the situations where minor surgery might pose a risk or might be contraindicated. Tables 3 and 4 summarise the precautions and contraindications of MS in Primary Care.

• Diabetes mellitus and peripheral vascular disease when planning surgery in the lower extremities
• In patients with chronic use of immunosuppressors (corticosteroids)
• Do not add vasoconstrictor to local anaesthetic in patients with arrhythmia, severe hypertension, hyperthyroidism, pheochromocytoma, pregnancy and in anaesthesia of the fingers
• Anatomic areas of risk (Figure 8 A and 8B)
• Research specifies the use of oral anticoagulants and antiplatelet since we must raise the suppression (assess risk-benefit) prior to the surgery. Currently, Holbrook et al [36] considered that these patients can be operated without changing its pattern whether taking oral anticoagulants (if your INR is within the therapeutic range) as antiplatelet
• *Specific precautions with the use of electrocautery:* Keep the patient's skin clear from any metallic object (metal dentures, implants, prosthesis and IUD are not contraindicated), Do not use alcohol or use the bovie near a source of oxygen . Use latex gloves for insulation
• *Special precautions for cryosurgery:* Patients with areas of potential circulatory compromise due to the risk of necrosis. Hairy areas in which hair loss could ensue. Hyperpigmented areas (black or dark skin) where the use of cryosurgery can leave areas of hypopigmentation. Patients with high levels of cryoglobulins.

Table 3. Precautions of MS in family medicine

• Unless justified exceptions, never involve, malignant skin lesions in family medicine. Likewise, if the pathological result of lesion excised is malignant, should be performed interconsultation with other specialists.
• Allergy to local anaesthetics.
• Pregnancy: we must postpone the surgery, and if malignancy is suspected, refer to the appropriate specialist.
• Acute intercurrent disease: will be postponed until recovery.
• Doubts about the motivations of the patient: surgery is contraindicated in patients whose motivation for it is questionable or if there is excessive preoccupation with the aesthetic result
• In patients with severe psychiatric disorders or uncooperative patients is contraindicated performing MS in family medicine.
• Refusal to any activity reported minor surgical consent.

Table 4. Contraindications of MS in family medicine

8.1.1. Pre-medication

In the case of patients who are anxious about the intervention, we can consider pre-operatory sedation and can use diazepam 5–10 mg oral or sublingual or lorazepam 1–5 mg sublingual, administered 30 minutes prior to the intervention.

8.2. Intra-operatory complications

A vasovagal syncope is the most frequent form of complication and is common in young males. Treatment consists of placing the patient in the Trendelenburg position, administering oxygen

http://dx.doi.org/10.5772/62650

and fluid therapy, and if it is deemed necessary, the use of atropine can be considered: 0.5–1 mg SC or IV (maximum 2 mg). In general, the majority of episodes recover spontaneously after a few seconds or a few minutes.

In centres where programmed MS is carried out, it is obligatory to always have CPR cardio-pulmonary resuscitation (CPR)materials and medication to hand (as previously indicated).

8.3. Post-operatory complications

Table 5 lists the complications that might appear following an MS intervention.

• **Hematoma-seroma**: To prevent their formation, a correct intraoperative hemostasis is paramount plus suturing the wound in layers with no gaps and, finally, applying a compressive bandage.
• **Infection**: Can occur in up to 1% of minor surgical patients and it appears as swelling, redness of the wound edges and, sometimes, purulent discharge. Symptoms such as fever and / or chills are only rarely seen. Infections are treated by removing some of the stitches, plus daily cleaning and disinfection of the wound and allowing the wound to close by secondary intention. If necessary, a drain may be inserted into the wound and an oral antibiotic regimen may be initiated.
• **Wound dehiscence**: The separation of the edges of the wound before proper healing. There are predisposing factors secondary to surgery (excessive tension on the edges of the wound, use of inappropriate suture material or early suture withdrawal) or it may be the final phase of other complications such as hematoma or infection. After wound dehiscence, wound repair will take place by secondary intention, resulting in a poor cosmetic result.
• **Hypertrophic scar and keloid**: are very difficult to prevent and their most frequent location is in the chest, shoulders and upper back, in young people and blacks. Treatment of these scars is difficult and results are often discouraging. Occlusive treatment or steroid injections may be tried.

Table 5. Postoperative complications in MS

Author details

José María Arribas Blanco[1*], Shabnan Habibi[2], Nuria Rodríguez Pata[2] and José Ramón Castello Fortet[3]

*Address all correspondence to: jarribasb@gmail.com

1 Family Medicine, Faculty of Medicine, Autonomous University of Madrid, Madrid, Spain

2 Family Medicine, University Health Center "Cerro del Aire" Majadahonda, Madrid, Spain

3 Plastic and Reconstructive Surgery, University Hospital "Clínica Puerta de Hierro", Madrid, Spain

[1,2,3] Members of Grupo de Trabajo de Cirugía Menor en Medicina de Familia

References

[1] Arribas JM. Cirugía menor y procedimientos en medicina de familia (2ª edición). 2006 Madrid: Jarpyo Editores, ISBN 84-96549-05-4 (vol I): 84-96549-04-6 (vol II. III y IV).

[2] Programa formativo de la especialidad de Medicina Familiar y Comunitaria. Comisión Nacional de la Especialidad de Medicina Familiar y Comunitaria. Ministerio de Sanidad y Consumo - Ministerio de Educación y Ciencia. Madrid (España), 17 de enero de 2005

[3] Van Dijk CE, Verheij RA, Spreeuwenberg P, Groenewegen PP, de Bakker DH. Minor surgery in general practice and effects on referrals to hospital care: observational study. BMC Health Serv Res. 2011;11:2 http://www.ncbi.nlm.nih.gov/pubmed/21205305

[4] George S, Pockney P, Primrose J, Smith H, Little P, Kinley H, Kneebone R, Lowy A, Leppard B, Jayatilleke N, McCabe C. A prospective randomised comparison of minor surgery in primary and secondary care. The MiSTIC trial. Health Technol Assess. 2008 May; 12(23):iii-iv, ix-38. http://www.ncbi.nlm.nih.gov/pubmed/18505669

[5] O'Cathain A, Brazier JE, Milner PC, Fall M. Cost effectiveness of minor surgery in general practice: a prospective comparison with hospital practice. Br J Gen Pract 1992;42:13–17. http://www.ncbi.nlm.nih.gov/pubmed/1586525

[6] Arribas JM. Pasado, presente y futuro de la cirugía menor en Atención Primaria. Artículo editorial. Aten Primaria 2011; 43(2):58–60. http://www.ncbi.nlm.nih.gov/pubmed/21353148

[7] Davis CR, Toll EC, Bates AS, Cole MD, Smith FC. Surgical and procedural skills training at medical school - a national review. Int J Surg. 2014. pii: S1743-9191(14)00168-X. http://www.ncbi.nlm.nih.gov/pubmed/24909137

[8] Delaney EK, Duckworth L, Thompson WD, Lee AJ, Murchie P. Excising squamous cell carcinomas: comparing the performance of GPs, hospital skin specialists and other hospital specialists. Fam Pract. 2012;29(5):541–546. http://www.ncbi.nlm.nih.gov/pubmed/22321614

[9] Hansen C, Wilkinson D, Hansen M, Soyer HP. Factors contributing to incomplete excision of non melanoma skin cancer by Australian general practitioners. Arch Dermatol. 2009;145(11):1253–1260. http://www.ncbi.nlm.nih.gov/pubmed/19917954

[10] Bakhai M, Hopster D, Wakeel R. A retrospective study comparing the accuracy of prehistology diagnosis and surgical excision of malignant melanomas by general practitioners and hospital specialists. Clin Exp Dermatol. 2010;35(1):63–67. http://www.ncbi.nlm.nih.gov/pubmed/19778304

[11] Pockney P, Primrose J, George S, Jayatilleke N, Leppard B, Smith H, Little P, Kneebone R and Lowy A. Recognition of skin malignancy by general practitioners: obser-

vational study using data from a population-based randomised controlled trial. Br J Cancer. 2009 ;100(1):24–27. http://www.ncbi.nlm.nih.gov/pubmed/19127264

[12] Arribas JM, Hernández M. Skills in Minor Surgical Procedures for General Practitioners. In: O. Capelli (Ed.), Primary Care at a Glance – Hot Topics and New Insights, 2012. ISBN 978-953-51-0539-8.

[13] Pfenninger JL, Fowler GC. Procedures for Primary Care, 3rd ed. 2011. Elsevier-Mosby: St Louis, Missouri. ISBN: 978-0323052672

[14] Tanner J, Swarbrook S, Stuart J. Surgical hand antisepsis to reduce surgical site infection. Cochrane DatabaseSyst Rev. 2008;(1):CD004288. doi: 10.1002/14651858.CD004288.pub2. http://www.ncbi.nlm.nih.gov/pubmed/18254046

[15] Czarnowski C, Ponka D, Rughani R, Geoffrion P. See one. Do one. Teach one: office-based minor surgical procedures. Can Fam Physician. 2008;54(6):893. http://www.ncbi.nlm.nih.gov/pubmed/18556500

[16] Zuber TJ. Punch biopsy of the skin. Am Fam Physician. 2002;65(6):1155–1158, 1161–1162, 1164. http://www.aafp.org/afp/2002/0315/p1155.html

[17] Freiman A, Bouganim N. History of cryotherapy. Dermatol Online J. 2005;11(2):9. http://www.ncbi.nlm.nih.gov/pubmed/16150217

[18] Hainer BL. Electrosurgery for the skin. Am Fam Physician. 2002;66(7):1259–1266. http://www.ncbi.nlm.nih.gov/pubmed/12387438

[19] Kudur MH, Pai SB, Sripathi H, Prabhu S. Sutures and suturing techniques in skin closure. Indian J Dermatol Venereol Leprol. 2009;75(4):425–434. http://www.ncbi.nlm.nih.gov/pubmed/19584482

[20] Moy RL, Lee A, Zalka A. Commonly used suturing techniques in skin surgery. Am Fam Physician. 1991;44(5):1625–1634. http://www.ncbi.nlm.nih.gov/pubmed/1950960

[21] Iavazzo C, Gkegkes ID, Vouloumanou EK, Mamais I, Peppas G, Falagas ME. Sutures versus staples for the management of surgical wounds: a meta-analysis of randomized controlled trials. Am Surg. 2011; 77(9):1206–1221. http://www.ncbi.nlm.nih.gov/pubmed/21944632

[22] Coulthard P, Esposito M, Worthington HV, van der Elst M, van Waes OJ, Darcey J. Tissue adhesives for closure of surgical incisions. Cochrane Database Syst Rev. 2010;(5):CD004287. doi: 10.1002/14651858.CD004287.pub3. http://www.ncbi.nlm.nih.gov/pubmed/20464728

[23] Singer AJ, Quinn JV, Hollander JE. The cyanoacrylate topical skin adhesives. Am J Emerg Med. 2008;26(4):490–496. http://www.ncbi.nlm.nih.gov/pubmed/18410821

[24] Tajirian AL, Goldberg DJ.A review of sutures and other skin closurematerials. J Cosmet Laser Ther. 2010;12(6):296–302. doi: 10.3109/14764172.2010.538413. http://www.ncbi.nlm.nih.gov/pubmed/21142740

[25] Hochberg J, Meyer KM, Marion MD. Suture choice and other methods of skin closure. Surg Clin North Am. 2009; 89 (3):627–641. http://www.ncbi.nlm.nih.gov/pubmed/19465201

[26] Castelló JR, Arribas JM, Fernández-Cañadas S. Procedimientos de corte e incisiones quirúrgicas. En: Arribas JM. Cirugía menor y procedimientos en medicina de familia (2ª edición). 2006 Madrid: Jarpyo Editores, ISBN 84-96549-05-4 (vol I): 84-96549-04-6 (vol II. III y IV).

[27] Zuber TJ. Fusiform excision. Am Fam Physician. 2003;67(7):1539–1544, 1547–1548, 1550.

[28] Phelps RG, Lebwohl MG. Biopsy techniques: shave, punch, or excision? JAMA Dermatol. 2014; 150(1):12–13. http://www.ncbi.nlm.nih.gov/pubmed/24285132

[29] Pickett H. Shave and punch biopsy for skin lesions. Am Fam Physician. 2011;84(9): 995–1002. http://www.ncbi.nlm.nih.gov/pubmed/22046939

[30] Castelló JR, Arribas JM, Sánchez Olaso A. Procedimientos de sutura quirúrgica. En: Arribas JM. Cirugía menor y procedimientos en medicina de familia (2ª edición). 2006 Madrid: Jarpyo Editores, ISBN 84-96549-05-4 (vol I): 84-96549-04-6 (vol II. III y IV)

[31] Edlich RF, Gubler K, Wallis AG, Clark JJ, Dahlstrom JJ, Long WB.Scientific basis for the selection of skin closure techniques. J Environ Pathol Toxicol Oncol. 2010;29(4): 363–372. http://www.ncbi.nlm.nih.gov/pubmed/21284598

[32] Zuber TJ. The mattress sutures: vertical, horizontal, and corner stitch. Am Fam Physician. 2002;66(12):2231–2236. http://www.ncbi.nlm.nih.gov/pubmed/12507160

[33] Avilés JA, Lázaro P. Prognosis for cutaneous melanoma according to surgical department: comparative study at a tertiary care hospital. Actas Dermosifiliogr. 2006;97(4): 247–252. http://www.ncbi.nlm.nih.gov/pubmed/16801017

[34] McKenna DB, Marioni JC, Lee RJ, Prescott RJ, Doherty VR. A comparison of dermatologists', surgeons' and general practitioners' surgical management of cutaneous melanoma. Br J Dermatol. 2004;151(3):636–644 http://www.ncbi.nlm.nih.gov/pubmed/15377351

[35] Kraft J, Murray CA. The fusiform skin excision: one recipe for success. J Cutan Med Surg. 2011;15(5):245–249. http://www.ncbi.nlm.nih.gov/pubmed/21962182

[36] Holbrook A, Schulman S, Witt DM, et al. Evidence-based management of anticoagulant therapy: antithrombotic therapy and prevention of thrombosis, 9th ed: American College of Chest Physicians evidence-based clinical practice guidelines. Chest. 2012;141(suppl2):e152S–e184S. doi: 10.1378/chest.11-2295 http://www.ncbi.nlm.nih.gov/pubmed/22315259

Chapter 7

Allergic Sensitization in Rhinitis and Asthma

Eleonora Savi, Silvia Peveri and Oreste Capelli

Additional information is available at the end of the chapter

http://dx.doi.org/10.5772/63009

Abstract

Allergic rhinitis (AR) is usually defined as an inflammatory disease of the nasal mucosa induced by an interaction of environmental allergens and IgE in sensitized patients. Its symptoms are sneezing, nasal itching, rhinorrhoea and nasal obstruction. Allergic rhinitis affects approximately 20- 30% of the population worldwide and its prevalence is increasing. Isolated AR is rare and it actually has to be considered as a systemic allergic disease, associated to comorbidities, such as conjunctivitis, chronic middle ear effusions, irregular sleep, sinusitis, lymphoid hypertrophy with obstructive sleep apnoea. The most relevant comorbidity is asthma, a heterogeneous disease, usually characterized by chronic airway inflammation in which many cells and cellular elements play an important role. Bronchial asthma is characterized by bronchial hyper-reactivity and symptoms may be triggered or worsened by factors such as viral infections, allergens, tobacco smoke, exercise and stress. A state of "minimal persistent inflammation" is permanently maintained in the lower respiratory tract of asthmatic individuals. The diagnosis of asthma is based on evidence of variable airflow limitation tested with spirometry and a positive bronchodilation reversibility test. Skin prick tests (SPTs) are widely used to demonstrate an immediate IgE-mediated allergic reaction. They represent a major diagnostic tool in the field of allergy. Skin prick tests have a high specificity and sensitivity for the diagnosis of inhalant allergens. Immunotherapy (AIT) for allergic diseases has entered in a new age characterized by the development of a few innovative therapeutic classes of standardized allergen formulations registered. Clinical randomized trials have demonstrated the efficacy of AIT in allergic rhinitis in children and in adults, expressed in terms of reduction of symptom score and use of rescue medication. The efficacy is confirmed both for subcutaneous (SCIT) and sublingual (SLIT) immunotherapy in adults and in pediatric patients. The long lasting effect of AIT after its discontinuation is an important added value of this therapy. Controlled studies are available, where the carry-over effect of AIT is demonstrated for two years after discontinuance. The capacity to prevent new sensitizations, and to modify the evolution of the disease from the rhinitis to asthma are two important features of AIT. Allergen immunotherapy showed preventive capacity and also a carryover effect once treatment is discontinued.

Keywords: Rhinitis, asthma, allergy diagnostic, specific immunotherapy

INTECH
open science | open minds

© 2016 The Author(s). Licensee InTech. This chapter is distributed under the terms of the Creative Commons Attribution License (http://creativecommons.org/licenses/by/3.0), which permits unrestricted use, distribution, and reproduction in any medium, provided the original work is properly cited.

1. Introduction

Allergic rhinitis (AR) is an inflammatory disease of the nasal mucosa induced by allergens in sensitized patients with specific immunoglobulin E (IgE).

Its symptoms include sneezing, nasal itching, rhinorrhoea and nasal obstruction. Epidemiologically, AR represents a health problem for both children and adults on a global basis: approximately 20–30% of the population worldwide suffer its affects and its prevalence is increasing.

Genetic and socio-environmental factors may influence the development of AR: the urbanization processes, high levels of motor engine pollution and western lifestyles are significantly linked to high incidences of respiratory allergy diseases. Allergic rhinitis is not considered to be a serious disease but it significantly limits daily life activities, such as school and work performance – this leads to increased direct social costs (i. e., medical costs, mainly related to symptomatic medications) and indirect costs due to decreased work performance (AR is in fact one of the most significant causes of absenteeism from work).

The guidelines ARIA introduced for the first time represented a classification of severity of two degrees, according to the presence or absence of the effects of rhinitis on general well-being and quality of life (HRQL) and a classification regarding the duration of symptoms: "intermittent" and "persistent".

One component part of the symptoms of AR is nasal obstruction –the most disabling symptom as it seriously affects quality of life by interfering with normal sleep structures and over time facilitates the onset of complications such as allergic conjunctivitis, rhino-sinusitis and nasal polyposis, otitis media, adenoid hypertrophy and orthodontic problems.

The most relevant comorbidity is asthma. Past observations about the link between upper and lower airway disease has generated a united airway disease (UAD) notion. Around 38% of all AR patients present asthma symptoms or show a higher frequency of bronchial hyper-reactivity. In addition, 78% of asthma patients present rhinitis symptoms.

Allergic rhinitis can be considered a risk factor for asthma exacerbation. In asthmatic patients, AR symptoms induce worsened asthma control, more frequent asthma attacks and admission to emergency rooms; in addition the use of drugs for asthma significantly increases with the severity of AR. Diagnosis of asthma is based on evidence of a variable airflow limitation which is tested via spirometry and a positive bronchodilation reversibility test. Another test used to diagnose asthma is airways responsiveness: it is necessary in this test to measure how airways react when they are challenged with a trigger. Airway inflammation may also be tested via measurement of exhaled nitric oxide concentration. Nitric oxide is physiologically produced by lungs, but higher than normal levels indicate airways are inflamed, a condition which is associated with asthma.

The concordance of a typical history of allergic symptoms and the results of proper diagnostic tests forms the basis for AR diagnosis.

http://dx.doi.org/10.5772/63009

Skin prick tests (SPTs) are usually considered the standard diagnostic procedure to support an allergic basis for the patient's symptoms, to confirm suspected causes of the patient's symptoms and/or to identify sensitizing allergens.

The SPT represents the first line approach, to be preferred to *in vitro* IgE determination due to its high sensitivity, rapidity of performance, simplicity, ease of use and low cost.

International (EAACI, WAO) and national guidelines (SIAAIC) considered *in vitro* tests for allergic diseases as second-level tests, to be used after a SPT, for confirmation or in cases when an SPT cannot be carried out. Specific IgE for inhalant allergens (dust mites, dermatophagoides pteronyssinus, dermatophagoides farinae , pollens, latex, molds) and for some food allergens that can induce respiratory symptoms, are measured to understand trigger agents of allergic diseases such as conjunctivitis, rhinitis, asthma or professional allergic respiratory diseases.

This assay allows identification, in a quantitative way, of the sensitization towards a complete allergen and/or a specific allergy molecule. The possibility of performing a deeper analysis with molecular diagnostics gives important information which is more specific than from an SPT.

The identification of specific IgE against cross reacting molecules such as Profilins, Bet v1-PR10, lipid transfer protein and calcium-binding protein, or against "genuine molecules", represents an added value and allows distinction between true and false polysensitizations. Component resolved diagnosis has an important impact on the management of the patient in terms of the accuracy of the diagnosis, or the decision on therapies like specific immunotherapy prescription.

Immunotherapy for allergic diseases (AIT) has entered a new age, characterized by the development of a few innovative therapeutic classes of standardized, registered allergen formulations. AIT is considered a safe and efficacious treatment for patients with type-1 respiratory allergies. The ability of sublingual immunotherapy (SLIT) to elicit antigen specific tolerance is linked to the peculiar biology of oral antigen-presenting cells. In the absence of danger signals, Langerhans cells, myeloid dendritic cells and the macrophages located in oral tissues or the tonsils are biased towards the induction of Th1 and IL 10 producing CD4+ regulatory T cells.

Clinical randomized trials have demonstrated the efficacy of AIT in AR in children and adults, expressed in terms of are duction in symptom scores and the use of rescue medication.

2. Allergic rhinitis and its comorbidities

Allergic rhinitis (AR) is usually defined as an inflammatory disease of the nasal mucosa induced by an interaction of environmental allergens and immunoglobulin E (IgE) in sensitized patients [1].

Allergic rhinitis is the most widespread type of non-infectious rhinitis. Its symptoms include sneezing, nasal itching, rhinorrhoea and nasal obstruction. Ocular signs, such as itching of the eyes, redness and tearing, occur in a large percentage of patients suffering from AR.

Epidemiologically, AR represents a health problem for both children and adults on a global basis. Allergic rhinitis affects approximately 20–30% of the population worldwide and its prevalence is increasing. In Italy it is estimated that 24% of the population suffers of AR (data 2007–2010 GEIRD-LIBRA) [2]. Nevertheless, around one-third of allergic patients have never visited a physician, an observation which suggests that the actual prevalence of AR may be underestimated with the condition perhaps being mistreated [3].

Allergic rhinitis is usually categorized as a multi-factorial disease and many hypothesis hypotheses have been suggested to explain its increasing occurrence.

As in case of asthma, genetic factors may influence the development of AR; these diseases reveal strong familial and intra-individual clustering, implying an overlapping disease aetiology.

A socio-environmental hypothesis is based on several studies, demonstrating that the urbanization process, high levels of motor engine pollution and western lifestyles are significantly linked to the high incidence of respiratory allergy diseases, found to prevail among inhabitants of metropolitan areas over rural areas [4].

Allergic rhinitis is not considered a serious disease and although it is certainly not life threatening it does significantly limit daily activities such as an individual's performance at school or work, which leads to increased direct social costs (i. e., medical costs, mainly related to symptomatic medications) and indirect costs due to a decrease in workforce performance (AR is in fact one of the most significant causes of absenteeism).

The guidelines ARIA introduced had for the first time a classification of severity of two degrees, according to the presence or absence of the effects of rhinitis on general well-being and on the quality of life (health-related quality of life, HRQL).

By means of a validated questionnaire, it has been possible to demonstrate that AR has a real and measurable impact on HRQL, considered more important than more serious, chronic diseases, such as diabetes mellitus. For a patient with AR, important limitations coexist, due directly to rhinitis symptoms and indirectly to chronic use of drugs –both can impact social life: e. g., sleep disorders leading to daytime sleepiness and increased accidents, difficulty in concentrating, headaches, mood changes, depression, irritability and fatigue. When considered altogether, these conditions can heavily weigh on a person's social and professional life [5].

As part of the symptoms of AR, nasal obstruction is the most disabling as it seriously affects quality of life by interfering with normal sleep patterns. It also facilitates the onset of complications such as rhino-sinusitis and nasal polyposis.

Allergic Rhinitis classification is based on both duration and chronicity as well as on the grading of severity (mild or moderate–severe) of symptoms. It also takes into account the impact of the disease on daily activities, such as work/school performance and impaired sleep.

Regarding duration of symptoms, AR is defined "intermittent" when it occurs less than 4 days per week or less than 4 consecutive weeks per year. Vice versa, "persistent" AR occurs when symptoms are present more than 4 days per week and more than 4 consecutive weeks per year.

Isolated AR is rare and it actually has to be considered as a systemic allergic disease, associated to comorbidities, such as conjunctivitis, chronic middle ear effusions, irregular sleep, sinusitis, lymphoid hypertrophy with obstructive sleep apnoea. However, the most relevant comorbidity is asthma. Past observations about the link between upper and lower airways disease has generated the notion of united airway disease (UAD) [6].

The relationship between the two compartments is clinical, epidemiological, functional and immunological. Subsequently, the official standpoint is that rhinitis is both allergic and non-allergic, and is acknowledged as a risk factor for asthma.

Recent surveys show that around 38% of all AR patients present asthma symptoms too. On the other hand, 78% of asthma patients present rhinitis symptoms.

This finding is based not only on epidemiological data but also on physiological evidence. In fact, patients with AR (even without asthma) show a higher frequency of bronchial hyper-reactivity. This could be linked to the duration of AR and the number of sensitizations of patients.

Furthermore, AR can be considered as risk factor for asthma exacerbation. In asthmatic patients, AR symptoms induce worsened asthma control, more frequent asthma attacks and admission to emergency rooms. In addition, the use of drugs for asthma significantly increase with the severity of AR.

Other comorbid disorders and links to AR, are:

a. **Allergic conjunctivitis,** resulting in conjunctival injection chemosis, itchy eyes and tearing. These symptoms have been observed in more than 75% of patients with AR caused by pollen. Moreover, patients sensitized to pollen report ocular symptoms more frequently than patients sensitized to house dust mites [7].

b. AR patients compared with non-allergic subjects are more frequently affected by **rhinosinusitis**. Infections of the ear and of the nasal and paranasal sinuses are conditions secondary to the obstruction of the Eustachian tube as a consequence of local inflammatory infiltrate [8]. Patients with AR, particularly those sensitized to house dust mites, rarely develop **nasal polyps** [9]. Some studies show that around 21% of AR patients are affected by **otitis media**. In the case of AR in children, the incidence of otitis media is twice as large when compared to non-allergic children [10].

c. It has been reported that among children with AR, particularly if sensitized to dust mites, **adenoid hypertrophy** (AH) occurs significantly more frequently than in children with other allergic diseases (asthma/atopic dermatitis) or without allergies. **Sleep and quality of life**: nasal obstruction resulting from rhinitis causes sleep disorders, fatigue and tiredness during the day, as well asloss of smell and taste [11]. Chronic nasal obstruction in children can cause excessive breathing through the mouth which leads to **orthodontic problems** such as an excessive stretching of the face and malocclusion.

The concordance of a typical history of allergic symptoms and the results of properdiagnostic tests formsthe basis of AR diagnosis.

Skin prick tests (SPTs) are usually considered the standard diagnostic procedure to support an allergic basis for the patient's symptoms, to confirm suspected causes of the patient's symptoms and/or to identify sensitizing allergens.

The reasons for preference of the SPT as a first line approach, over *in vitro* IgE determination are the following: high sensitivity, rapidity of performance, simplicity, ease of use and low cost.

Nonetheless, particular situations (extensive skin disease, skin test suppressive therapy, such as antihistamines that cannot be discontinued, or uncooperative patients) are indications for using serum specific IgE determination by immunoassays.

In some cases of rhinitis further study is useful via fibre optic nasal endoscopy, such as for a typical symptoms or physical findings, complications, other suspected conditions or when symptoms apparently do not respond to therapy. For suspected complications or comorbidities such as nasal polyposis with sinusitis, a computed tomography (CT) scan may be useful.

Before prescribing immunotherapy it is useful to study nasal cellularity via nasal cytology [12]. Cytological findings can in fact support the allergic pathogenesis of rinithis (neutrophil infiltration for mite allergy, eosinophilic infiltrate in the case of hay fever) or might indicate non-allergic rhinitis [13].

3. Asthma

Asthma is a heterogeneous disease, usually characterized by chronic airway inflammation in which many cells and cellular elements play an important role.

Chronic inflammation causes an associated increase in airway hyper-responsiveness leading to recurrent episodes of wheezing, breathlessness, chest tightness and coughing, particularly at night or in the early hours of the morning. Generally, these episodes are accompanied by widespread but variable airflow obstruction that is often reversible, either spontaneously or following therapy.

The pathogenesis of these alterations involves many mechanisms, in particular inflammatory cell infiltration, mediator release and airway remodelling.

As reported in the definition, bronchial asthma is characterized by bronchial hyper-reactivity, and its symptoms may be triggered, or worsened, by factors such as viral infections, allergens, tobacco smoke, exercise and stress. A state of "minimal persistent inflammation" is permanently maintained in the lower respiratory tract of asthmatic individuals. The intensity of clinical symptoms varies in relation to the actual size of the bronchial obstruction and to the degree of its subjective perception by the patient [14].

The probability that respiratory disease is really asthma becomes lower if the patient has:

- An isolated cough with no other respiratory symptoms. Chronic production of sputum. Shortness of breath associated with dizziness, light-headedness or peripheral tingling. Chest pain. Exercise-induced dyspnoea with noisy inspiration (stridor).

The diagnosis must be done preferably before starting treatment because it is often more difficult to confirm the diagnosis afterwards.

It is increasingly clear that bronchial asthma is not a single disease but a complex set of overlapping syndromes; for classification purposes it is necessary to take into account the phenotype of the disease resulting from a given set of genetic and environmental interactions.

In a recent review a classification has been proposed based on phenotypes of asthma which takes into account both clinical and physiological triggers as well as the cell types involved in inflammation.

From the clinical and physiological point of view it is necessary to classify asthma according to its severity; in order to define severity several parameters are considered: for instance, the frequency of exacerbations and age of onset correlate with a more favorable prognosis and improved lung function in the case of early-onset, typically allergic asthma; in contrast, resistance to drug treatment(especially neutrophilic asthma) and its possible association with chronic restriction is mainly observed in non-allergic patients.

As far as triggering factors are concerned, bronchial asthma should be further divided into allergic asthma, often associated with rhinitis and conjunctivitis but with a favorable prognosis; exercise-induced asthma; occupational asthma (about15% of asthma in adults); aspirin sensitive asthma (with eosinophilic inflammation and frequent association with nasal polyposis and sinusitis) and premenstrual asthma [15].

Finally, asthma should be characterized according to the specific cellularity responsible for inflammation in eosinophilic or neutrophilic. It is increasingly clear that the correct identification of phenotype of asthma is essential to set a targeted therapy and to obtain good control of symptoms and improve the quality of life of patients [16]. The classification of severity of asthma is assessed retrospectively from the level of treatment required to control symptoms and exacerbations:

- Mild asthma: well controlled with as needed relief medication alone or with a low dose of inhaled corticosteroids (ICS), leukotriene receptor antagonist or cromones.
- Moderate asthma: well controlled with a low dose of ICS/long-acting beta agonist (LABA).
- Severe asthma: controlled with high dose ICS/LABA or asthma that remains uncontrolled despite this treatment. In the diagnosis of severe asthma it is important to exclude common causes of uncontrolled asthma such as poor inhaler technique, poor medication adherence, incorrect diagnosis of asthma, comorbidities (rhinosinusitis, gastroesophageal reflux, obesity, obstructive sleep apnoea).

Asthma can be effectively treated and when asthma is well-controlled, patients can avoid troublesome symptoms during the day and night, need little or no relief medication, have productive, physically active lives, normal lung function and avoid serious exacerbations.

The diagnosis of asthma is based on evidence of variable airflow limitation tested with spirometry and a positive bronchodilation reversibility test [17].

The spirometry allows to two main measurements: the volume of air that the patient can exhale in the first second of exhalation (the forced expiratory volume in one second, or FEV_1] and the total amount of air that the patient blows out (the forced vital capacity or FVC). These readings are compared against the average measurements for people of the same age, sex and height, and immediately indicate if airways are obstructed or not. The most important spirometric value is the FVC. To measure FVC, the patient inhales maximally, and then exhales as rapidly and as completely as possible. Normal lungs generally can empty more than 80%of their volume in 6 seconds or less. The forced expiratory volume in one second (FEV_1] is the volume of air exhaled in the first second of the FVC maneuver. The FEV_1/FVC ratio is expressed as a percentage and is known as the Tiffeneau Index. A reduced value of FEV_1 and of absolute FEV_1/FVC ratio indicates an obstructive ventilatory pattern. In this case, a bronchodilator challenge test is recommended to detect patients with reversible airway obstruction. This is known as "reversibility testing", and it can be useful in distinguishing asthma from other lung pathological conditions, such as chronic obstructive pulmonary disease (COPD).

Another test used to diagnose asthma is airway responsiveness. When the diagnosis is not possible from the above described test it is necessary to measure how airways react when they are challenged with a trigger. The test involves inhaling progressively increasing amounts of a medication (e. g., metacholine, histamine) at regular intervals, and taking FEV_1 measurements to see if they fall below a certain threshold (typically 80% of baseline values). In some cases, exercise may be used as a trigger.

Testing airway inflammation may also be useful. This can be done by measuring the exhaled nitric oxide concentration. Nitric oxide is physiologically produced by the lungs, but higher than normal levels indicate airways are inflamed, a condition which is associated with asthma [18].

4. Allergy diagnostics *in vivo*: when, what, who?

The SPT is widely used to demonstrate an immediate IgE-mediated allergic reaction. These tests represent a major diagnostic tool in the field of allergy. Skin prick tests have a high specificity and sensitivity for the diagnosis of inhalant allergens.

Their simplicity, rapidity of performance, low cost, and high sensitivity explain their key position in the diagnosis of allergies. If properly performed, they yield useful evidence for the diagnosis of a specific allergy. In respiratory allergies skin tests represent the first diagnostic method used in patients with a suggestive clinical history of allergic rhinitis, conjunctivitis and/or asthma. They can be used from infancy to old age [19].

Usually, skin tests are performed on one or both forearms, depending on the age and size of the patient. SPTs can be performed and interpreted in infants; usually the size of the lower arm limits the number of allergens that can be tested. Prick testing involves introducing a needle into the upper layers of the skin and releasing a drop of allergen extract after gently lifting the epidermis. The release of preformed histamine from mast cells causes increased vascular permeability via smooth muscle contraction and development of a wheal; inflammatory mediators initiate a neural reflex causing vasodilatation, leading to erythema (the flare). The distance between two prick tests should be 2 cm to avoid cross-contamination [20]. It is important to avoid bleeding of the skin. Negative (saline) and positive (e. g., 9% histamine hydrochloride solution) controls are required in SPTs to make any interpretation possible. The positive control should optimally show a wheal diameter of ‡3 mm [21].

Skin tests are regarded positive if the mean wheal diameter is ≥3 mm. Very large reactions are not necessarily associated with a more severe disease. Skin test results may be negative even if patients are allergic. If a skin test is positive, one will have to distinguish reactions which are clinically relevant from those which are not. History and/or challenge tests help to clarify the relevance of a sensitization. Usually, a clinically irrelevant sensitization does not lead to practical consequences.

Drugs can suppress skin tests, therefore, it is always necessary to ask patients about the medication they have taken in the preceding days. This is particularly the case for oral H1-antihistamines [22], but I also the case for anxiolytics –not however for antidepressants [23]. Topical skin corticosteroids may also alter skin reactivity. The inhibitory effect of H1-antihistamines lasts about 2–7 days while the inhibitory effect of topical steroids lasts up to 7 days.

False-positive skin tests may result from dermographism, 'irritant' reactions or a non-specific enhancement from a nearby strong reaction. Contamination of the needle by another allergen extract may also induce false-positive results. To overcome this problem, it is recommended that needles or puncture devices be changed between each test.

False-negative skin tests can be caused by poor potency of extracts [24], drugs modulating the allergic reaction, diseases attenuating the skin's response, weak punctures or a limited local production of allergen-specific IgE– only in the nose [25] or eyes [26].

Inhalant allergens to be tested should be chosen after considering various factors: the spread environment, the homologies between the various pollen and lifestyle habits. The Global Allergy and Asthma European Network suggested a panel of allergens to be tested in all patients in Europe: Pollen (Birch, Cypress, Grass, Mugwort, Olive, Parietaria officinalis, Ragweed), house dust mites, animals (dog and cat) and moulds (Alternaria, Cladosporium).

The SPT is usually considered to be a safe procedure, but recently there have been occasional reports of generalized allergic reactions or vasovagal reactions [27]. Based on the literature, the occurrence of systemic reactions with inhalant allergens has diminished over the last 30years. In general, the risk of systemic reactions is lower with SPTs than with intradermal testing. Some patients (those with histories of previous anaphylactic reactions, small children, pregnant women, uncontrolled asthmatic sand those with a high degree of reactivity) should be considered at higher risk of systemic/anaphylactic reactions. Based on the literature, the risk of fatality due to an SPT is extremely remote, and severe/anaphylactic reactions are rare. Nevertheless, this risk cannot be completely excluded, especially in highly susceptible subjects. Physicians who perform SPTs should be aware of this and apply simple precautionary rules [28].

5. Allergy diagnostics *in vitro*: few appropriate allergens

Specific IgE can be detected either *in vivo* by SPTs or *in vitro* by specific IgE assay: both methods usually employ whole extracts from allergenic sources which contain a mixture of allergenic and non-allergenic proteins [29] –the IgE response is specifically directed towards some molecules [30]. Specific IgE for inhalant allergens (dust mites, dermatophagoides pteronyssinus, dermatophagoides farinae, pollens, latex, molds) and for some food allergens that can induce respiratory symptoms (serum albumin, wheat flour, casein, fish parvalbumin, vegetables as Lipid Transfer Protein, lysozyme, etc.) are measured to understand the trigger agents of allergic diseases such as conjunctivitis, rhinitis, asthma or professional allergic respiratory diseases.

International (EAACI European Allergy Asthma Clinical immunology, WAO World Allergy Organization) and National Guidelines (SIAAIC Società italiana Asma Allergia Immunologia Clinica) considered *in vitro* tests for allergic diseases as a second-level test, to be used after the SPT, for confirmation or in the case where the SPT cannot be carried out because the patient takes antihistamine drug so r shows atopic dermatitis, etc.

Measurement of *in vitro* specific IgE (sIgE) is an important tool.

It allows the identification, in a quantitative way, of the sensitization towards a complete allergen and/or a specific allergy molecule. The possibility to perform a deeper analysis with molecular diagnostics gives important information, more specific than that gained from the SPT. Specific IgE is usually measured for common allergens: dermatophagoides, grass, trees, cypress, pellitory, ragweed, plantagolanceolata, olive pollen, alternaria, dog and cat dander and cladosporium herbarum with particular concern to botanicals.

Extractive preparations used for SPTs usually contain cross-reactive components which are highly conserved across widely different allergen sources [31]. This may complicate the interpretation of the diagnostic results, especially in polysensitized subjects. The introduction of highly purified natural and recombinant single allergenic molecules represents an important improvement in the diagnosis of IgE sensitizations and cross reactivities.

6. Component resolve diagnostics

The identification of a specific IgE against cross-reacting molecules such as Profilins, Bet v1-PR10, lipid transfer protein, calcium-binding protein or against "genuine molecules", represents an added value and allows the distinction between true and false polysensitizations. A true polysensitization occurs when specific IgE is present against genuine components of different allergenic sources. The genuine molecules for grass sensitization are: Phl p1, usually the first allergen of grass induces IgE and Phl p 5; Bet v 1, is the genuine molecule of birch, Par j2 of Pellitory, Pla l 1 of Plantago l, Amb a 1 of ragweed, Fe d1 of cat, Der p 1 and Der p 2 of Dermathophagoides are the genuine molecules of dust mites. False polysensitizations are due to the presence of panallergens like profilin or calcium-binding proteins causing SPT positive results [32].

http://dx.doi.org/10.5772/63009

Component resolved diagnosis (CRD) has an important impact on the management of the patient in terms of the accuracy of the diagnosis, or decision on therapy (like specific immunotherapy prescription). Recent studies [33] demonstrated that CRD use in the diagnostic pathway implies a change in the decision regarding treatment in more than 50% of patients compared to diagnosis based only on clinical history and skin test results [34].

An *in vitro* test is useful in these cases:

- *Positive SPT is in agreement with clinical history –in this case in vitro tests add information* [35] and allows: Detect of patients with sensitization to genuine molecules that cause allergic diseases [2]. Distinction among patients with positive prick tests for more than one allergen, about70% of allergic patients have a polysensitization due to sensitization to pan-allergens [36, 37]. Evaluate in childhood of the "spreading" of sensitization towards each grass molecule and has prognostic information about the evolution of the disease: a correlation between phenotypes of sensitization and illness severity [38, 39, 40]. Choice of better therapies: if only clinical history and prick tests are used, without the support of CRD results, the choice of the therapy is incorrect in more than 50% of the cases, with an important cost increase [41, 42, 43]. Identification of the ideal patient for immunotherapy, represented by the patients with sensitization towards genuine molecules [44, 45] with high possibilities of improving symptoms and increasing safety during administration. Improvement to quality of life of allergic patients via the correct diagnosis [32]. Detection of patients with sensitization to pan-allergens such as *profilin* or *calcium-binding protein*. This can induce cross-reactivity with foods and pollens. Additionally, symptoms are shown for a long period of time if pollen grains are not detected in the air: the profilin, a molecule from grass, trees, ragweed pollen is able to induce nasal and bronchial inflammation for a long time period [34]. Management of the risk of anaphylaxis for allergic latex patients: it is important to detect IgE for latex molecules inducing anaphylaxis like Hev b 1, Hev b 3, Hev b 5, Hevb 6, to predict the risk of anaphylaxis; patients with only IgE for Hev b8 are not able to develop anaphylaxis because Hev b8 is not present in the surgery devices.
- *Negative prick tests and clinical history suitable for allergies: when there is not agreement between prick test results and clinical history*. Sometimes prick tests are less sensitivity than *in vitro* tests because the extract used for prick tests could miss some important allergenic molecules. *In vitro* tests can identify IgE towards particular molecules that induce allergic professional reactions: serum albumin, lipid transfer protein, lysozyme intake like preserves in some drugs, molecular allergens of Aspergillus like Asp f 4, Asp f6, Asp f 3 markers of Broncho-polmonar Aspergillosy or molecular allergens of Alternaria like the Alt a 1 marker of asthma [46, 47].

6.1. Allergen-specific immunotherapy can modify the natural history of allergies: The eligible patient

Immunotherapy for allergic diseases has entered a new age characterized by the development of a few innovative therapeutic classes of standardized, registered allergen formulations, which have been assigned marketing authorization codes (in Italy: AIC, Autorizzazioneall'Immissione in Commercio) as *bona fide* pharmaceutical specialties, having been supported by large and robust, randomized controlled clinical trials (RCT) [48].

The European Academy of Allergy Clinical Immunology EAACI and the American Academy of Allergic Asthma and Immunology (AAAI) has recently proposed the term "allergen immunotherapy" (AIT) to indicate the treatment of an allergic disease by a drug containing a given allergen.

To date, AIT products available on the market can be administered as sublingual immunotherapy (SLIT), but in principle subcutaneous immunotherapy (SCIT) products could be registered as well. AIT is considered a safe and efficacious treatment for patients with type-1 respiratory allergies [49, 1]. The ability of SLIT to elicit antigen-specific tolerance is linked to the peculiar biology of oral antigen-presenting cells. In the absence of danger signals, Langerhans cells, myeloid dendritic cells, macrophages located in oral tissues or tonsils are biased towards the inductions of Th 1 and IL 10 producing CD4+ regulatory T cells. This supports the induction of tolerance rather than an effector immune response generating inflammation. Sublingual administration does not lead to any detectable systemic exposure of intact allergens nor to the induction of new IgE sensitizations. Furthermore, due to the limited numbers of mast cells located in submucosal areas, SLIT has a very favorable safety profile, being adverse in its reaction locally and, only rarely systemically. The induction of CD4+ regulatory T cells and blocking anti-inflammatory IgGs or IgAs is considered important for tolerance induction after SLIT [50]. The clinical efficacy of AIT is supported by numerous clinical trials and meta-analyses [51].

6.1.1. Eligible patient for AIT

To identify the right patient to benefit from AIT the following criteria should be considered.

A) Proper diagnosis (IgE-mediated respiratory diseases).

B) Symptoms

- Rhinocongiuntivitis (rhinitis should be mild–severe persistent according to ARIA).
- Persistent symptoms for subjects responding poorly to medication. Interference with quality of life.
- Worsening of quality of life (sleep, social, working and school activities).
- Poor compliance to pharmacological therapy.
- Lack of comorbilities.

6.1.2. Clinical efficacy and disease-modifying effect

Clinical randomized trials have demonstrated the efficacy of AIT in AR in children and adults, expressed in terms of are duction of symptom score and use of rescue medication. The efficacy is confirmed both for subcutaneous (SCIT) and sublingual (SLIT) immunotherapy in adults and pediatric patients. AIT efficacy has been demonstrated with these allergenes: alternaria, grass, birch, pellitory, ragweed and Dermatophagoides.

In childhood SLIT is preferred to SCIT for patient compliance and safety.

The choice of SLIT or SCIT depends on several factors, including clinical conditions and risk–benefit evaluation. The long-lasting effect of AIT after its discontinuation is an important added value of this therapy as compared to pharmacological therapy. Controlled studies are available, where the carry-over effect of AIT is demonstrated, including the capacity to decrease symptom scores and rescue medication for two years after discontinuance. Previously, SLIT with non-registered products had been reported to maintain a favorable effect on patient respiratory allergies up to 12 years after discontinuation.

The capacity to prevent new sensitizations and to modify the evolution of the disease from rhinitis to asthma are two important features of AIT [52]. A trial which will formally evaluate the prevention of asthma with grass-based AIT is ongoing [53].

As part of acorrect allergic evaluation at baseline, the "asthma control test" (ACT), the "visual analog scale" (VAS) of symptoms, the results of spirometry and records of drug consumption should be completed before beginning AIT.

AIT is usually continued for 3–5 years. Patients undergoing this treatment should be controlled at least yearly and at the end of the treatment re-evaluated via ACT, VAS, spirometry and drug consumption.

Recent multicenter randomized double-blind studies with AIT in tablet form (registered drugs with AIC) demonstrated changes in the natural history of the disease.

The primary endpoint of this randomized controlled clinical study was to evaluate the efficacy of 75. 000 SQ grass tablets in patients with rhinoconjunctivitis to grass-based pollen. Major end-points were the score of rhinoconjunctivitis symptoms and symptomatic drug usage. The observation was extended not only to the 3 years of treatment but also to the 2 years of follow -up without therapy, in order to document the "disease modifying effect", according to the EMA's European Medicines Agency definition.

A total of 634 patients were randomized (1:1) to receive the tablet or placebo once a day.

The subjects had to receive the drug 4–8 months before the start of the grass pollen season.

The subjects in the active arm of this study had a symptoms score and drug usage of 31% and 21% lower than placebo, respectively.

If we also consider the weighted average of the combined score of symptoms and drug efficacy in the long term it is even more evident. The effect of the weighted mean score of symptoms and medications was 33%, and in each study year statistically significant results were observed. Some studies also included patients with mild and/or moderate asthma. In this case the combined weighted score for the symptoms of asthma was reduced by 39% compared to the placebo over the entire pollen season and 44% when taking into account only the peak of the pollen season. Importantly, a carry-over effect was observed both in the first and second year after the discontinuation of a 3-year treatment.

The treatment at the end of the fifth year (3 years of treatment and 2 years of follow-up without treatment) resulted in a statistically significant and clinically relevant 25% reduction (p = 0.

004) in the score of rhinoconjunctivitis symptoms, associated with a reduced usage of symptomatic drugs. In addition, the combined score of symptoms and medication showed a statistically significant reduction (-33%) on average for the 5 pollen seasons.

The efficacy of treatment was similar in monosensitized and polisensitized patients.

When considered together, these data confirm that AIT is capable of modifying the natural history of allergic with a carry-over effect which, being persistent for at least 2years after AIT discontinuation, can be considered "disease modifying" according to an EMA classification document [54].

6.1.3. Polisensitized patients

Epidemiological studies and clinical trials have shown that the percentage of polisensitization ranges from 20% to 90% with great variability depending on populations.

Polisensitization may also be associated with different clinical pictures with respect to monosensitized patients, especially those with a more impaired quality of life and more severe symptoms. In addition allergic children seem to display a higher frequency of sensitizations than their parents, especially in families with polisensitization. In addition, a small proportion of patients remain monosensitized during their whole lives. A functional defect of T-regulatory cells may explain the tendency to develop polisensitization. Children with persistent monosensitization produce higher amounts of Interleukin 10 and interferon gamma than children who develop polisensitization. This observation might envisage different immunologic phenotypes for monosensitizedand polisensitized patients [55]. While in North America AIT is composed of a mix of allergens, in Europe clinicians prefer to identify the most important allergen causing symptoms to choose AIT.

A series of real life multicentre observational studies named POLISMAIL (Polysensitization Impact on Immunotherapy) were conducted to elucidate the clinical relevance of polisensitization and were conducted in 11 allergy centers in Italy.

The POLISMAIL studies are based around several issues: polisensitization usually starts from childhood – polisensitization progresses with age for up to 80% of allergic adults – polisensitizationmay depend on a T-regulatory cell defect – polisensitization may significantly affect quality of life – polisensitizationmay be associated with more severe symptoms– polisensitization may discourage immunotherapy prescription.

The POLISMAIL studies indicated that polisensitization should not constitute an obstacle to AIT prescription. Only the clinically relevant allergens, such as the sensitizing allergen which is capable of inducing symptoms when inhaled, were chosen for AIT 56Some cases demonstrate true polisensitizations, other cases are sensitizations for pan allergens like profilin or calcium-binding proteins. Component resolve diagnosis (with either recombinant or purified allergens for prick tests or IgE in serum dosage) is a tool to improve the accurate identification of the sensitization allergens [57, 58]. A positive skin test could be a sensitization to a major allergen or simply be a result of a cross-reacting response to a panallergen like profilin Bet v 2 or Phl p 12, present with small conformational changes in both species of pollen. The demonstration of sensitization for genuine allergenic components and/or pan allergenic components can modify vaccine strategies [59].

6.1.4. AIT and quality of life

The aim of this position paper (the GA [2] LEN taskforce on patient reported outcomes (PROs) and health-related quality of life (HRQL)) is to define PROs and their meaning in asthma and rhinitis treatment, explore the available tools to provide criteria for a proper choice, identify patient-related factors which could influence PRO assessment, define specific recommendations for assessment, analysis and results spreading and underline unexplored areas and unmet needs. PROs assessment is gaining increasing importance, and it must be performed with a rigorous methodological procedure using validated tools. This approach enables a better understanding of patient-related factors influencing clinical trials and real-life management outcomes, identify patients subgroups that can benefit from specific treatment and management plans and tailor treatment to address PROs (not only physician-defined targets) to improve allergic asthma and rhinitis management and therapy. Allergic diseases can deeply interfere with patients' HRQL with detrimental effects to life being physical, psychological and social. Allergic rhinitis and asthma cause substantial social and economic burdens. School and work performance, including school and work absences, daily activity and quality of life are significantly impaired in both children and adults with respiratory allergies.

In order to measure if allergy disease modifies quality of life [60] many validated questionnaires are available. Most of them are specifically developed for AR, asthma and the evaluation of patients in AIT. HRQL has become an increasingly important aspect of outcome evaluation in healthcare research, providing a more comprehensive approach to patients, proving that nowadays we cannot renounce this tool [61].

International guidelines consider quality of life and other PROs an important primary outcome of clinical trials in order to evaluate the efficacy of AIT in allergic respiratory diseases ("Guideline on the clinical development of products for specific immunotherapy for the treatment of allergic diseases" 20 November 2008). Some variables could interfere with the results of PROs: age, stress, depression, coping, alessitimia. Clinical randomized trials show that AIT (SCIT and SLIT) improves quality of life and HRQL significantly [62, 63]).

6.1.5. Safety and tolerability

Clinical trials demonstrated that SLIT is generally safe and well tolerated in a real world setting. Usually adverse events are mild with rare and few severe reactions. Adverse reactions occur frequently during the first month of initiation or at the first administration: this confirms the importance of the first uptake being in the physician's office. Most of the patients show mild to moderate adverse reactions at the beginning of the treatment, however, the side effects tend to disappear after a few minutes. No fatal or near-fatal adverse reactions have been noticed [64]

6.1.6. AIT cost- effectiveness

The social costs of AR are very relevant and are estimated to be 4–6 billion dollars/year in the United States with average annual costs of 1089 euros per child and 1549 euros per adult in

Europe. The cost is higher if allergic asthma is included. Allergen immunotherapy showed a preventive capacity and also a carry-over effect once the treatment is discontinued.

International literature on the cost-effectiveness of immunotherapy for respiratory allergies included studies conducted based on an economic evaluation of AIT or allergic rhinoconjunctivitis, AR, asthma and rhinitis in combination with asthma. The evidence appears to support the cost-effectiveness of immunotherapy compared with pharmacotherapy for allergic rhinoconjunctivitis, and subcutaneous immunotherapy compared with pharmacotherapy for AR and asthma [65, 66].

The cost-effectiveness of immunotherapy depends on the duration of the clinical benefit of AIT following treatment discontinuance and on the break-even point of cumulative costs between immunotherapy and pharmacotherapy. This retrospective, and partly cross-sectional, study shows that high-dose sublingual immunotherapy may be effective in reducing the burden of disease as measured by the number of exacerbations need for medical visits and school–nursery time losses, with a considerable reduction of annual management costs. Also when considering only direct medical costs, the reduction is clear and appreciable when considering the whole population, as well as in the allergen type sub-samples and in the case-control sub-analysis of allergic asthmatic patients [67]. Patients with newly diagnosed AR initiating AIT incurred significantly in a lower healthcare costs than matched control subjects beginning 3 months after AIT initiation and continuing throughout the 18 month follow-up period. The significant cost benefits achieved by children with AR diagnoses who initiated AIT were also observed for adults with AR [68].

A prospective study demonstrated that SCIT was cost effectiveness after 6years of follow-up, in particular 3years after the drop of AIT [69]. The comparison of the cost of AIT and drug treatment must be discussed regarding the few available studies conducted in Germany and in the United states in the 1990s. Buchner reported in a retrospective, 10-year study that the direct and indirect costs in patients with AR and asthma were reduced by 54% in subjects treated with AIT compared with those treated with symptomatic drugs. Fisher estimated that the use of AIT could save respectively DM500 (610 dollars) and DM 1000 (1220 dollars) per year in subjects with AR and asthma. A recently retrospective study examined the economic effect of 3 years of AIT and a follow-up of 10 years: and found that the advantage ofdrug therapy started after 6 years.

Author details

Eleonora Savi[1*], Silvia Peveri[1] and Oreste Capelli[2]

*Address all correspondence to: e. savi@ausl. pc. it

1 Allergic Unit, G. da Saliceto Hospital, Piacenza, Italy

2 Clinical Governance Unit, Local Health Authority of Modena, Italy

References

[1] Bousquet J et al. Allergic Rhinitis and its Impact on Asthma (ARIA): achievements in 10 years and future needs. *J Allergy Clin Immunol*. 2012 Nov;130(5):1049–62.

[2] Scichilone N, Sanfilippo A, Sorino C, Giuliano L, Misseri M, Bellia V. Allergen sensitizations in southern Italy: a 5-year retrospective study in allergic respiratory patients. *Eur Ann Allergy Clin Immunol*. 2013 May;45(3):97–102.

[3] McMenamin P. Costs of hay fever in the United States in 1990. *Ann Allergy*. 1994; 73:35–9.

[4] Huang SK, Zhang Q, Qiu Z, Chung KF. Mechanistic impact of outdoor air pollution on asthma and allergic diseases. *J Thorac Dis*. 2015 Jan;7(1):23–33.

[5] Braido F, Baiardini I. Rhinasthma patient perspective: a short daily asthma and rhinitis QoL assessment. *Allergy*. 2012 Nov;67(11):1443–50.

[6] Compalati E, Ridolo E. The link between allergic rhinitis and asthma: the united airways disease. *Expert Rev Clin Immunol*. 2010 May;6(3):413–23.

[7] Gelardi M, Leo ME. Clinical characteristics associated with conjunctival inflammation in allergic rhinoconjunctivitis. *J Allergy Clin Immunol Pract*. 2015 Jan 26, S2213-2198(15)00011-2.

[8] Toppila-Salmi S. Molecular mechanisms of nasal epithelium in rhinitis and rhinosinusitis. *Curr Allergy Asthma Rep*. 2015 Feb;15(2):495.

[9] Gelardi M, Iannuzzi L, Tafuri S, Passalacqua G, Quaranta N. Allergic and non-allergic rhinitis: relationship with nasal polyposis, asthma and family history. *Acta Otorhinolaryngol Ital*. 2014 Feb;34(1):36–41.

[10] Quaranta N, Milella C, Iannuzzi L, Gelardi M. A study of the role of different forms of chronic rhinitis in the development of otitis media with effusion in children affected by adenoid hypertrophy. *Int J Pediatr Otorhinolaryngol*. 2013 Dec;77(12):1980–3.

[11] Chirakalwasan N, Ruxrungtham K. The linkage of allergic rhinitis and obstructive sleep apnea. *Asian Pac J Allergy Immunol*. 2014 Dec;32(4):276–86.

[12] Gelardi M. Seasonal changes in nasal cytology in mite-allergic patients. *J Inflamm Res*. 2014 Mar 28;7:39–44.

[13] Gelardi M. "Overlapped" rhinitis: a real trap for rhinoallergologists. *Eur Ann Allergy Clin Immunol*. 2014 Nov;46(6):234–6.

[14] Boulet LP, FitzGerald JM. A guide to the translation of the Global Initiative for Asthma (GINA) strategy into improved care. *Eur Respir J*. 2012 May;39(5):1220–9.

[15] Wenzel SE. Asthma: defining of the persistent adult phenotypes. *Lancet*. 2006 Aug 26;368(9537):804–13..

[16] Braido F, Baiardini I. Patients with asthma and comorbid allergic rhinitis: is optimal quality of life achievable in real life? *PLoS One*. 2012;7(2 e 31178).

[17] Bousquet J, Clark TJ. GINA guidelines on asthma and beyond. *Allergy*. 2007 Feb; 62(2):102–12.

[18] Dinh-Xuan AT. Contribution of exhaled nitric oxide measurement in airway inflammation assessment in asthma. A position paper from the French Speaking Respiratory Society. *Rev Mal Respir*. 2014 Nov 8.

[19] Demoly P, Bousquet J et al. Precision of skin prick and puncture tests with nine methods. *J Allergy Clin Immunol*. 1991 Nov;88(5):758–62.

[20] Piette V, Bourret E, Bousquet J, Demoly P. Prick tests to aeroallergens: is it possible simply to wipe the device between tests? *Allergy*. 2002;57:940–942.

[21] Bousquet J et al. Practical guide to skin prick tests in allergy to aeroallergens. *Allergy*. 2012 Jan;67(1):18.

[22] Simons FE. Advances in H1-antihistamines. *N Engl J Med*. 2004;351:2203–2217.

[23] Isik SR, Celikel S. The effects of antidepressants on the results of skin prick tests used in the diagnosis of allergic diseases. *Int Arch Allergy Immunol*. 2010;154:63–68.

[24] Dreborg S et al. Skin tests used in type I allergy testing. Position paper of the European academy of allergy and clinical immunology. *Allergy*. 1989;44(Suppl 10):1–69.

[25] Rondon C. Local IgE production and positive nasal provocation test in patients with persistent nonallergic rhinitis. *J Allergy Clin Immunol*. 2007;119:899–905.

[26] Leonardi A. Correlation between conjunctival provocation test (CPT) and systemic allergometric tests in allergic conjunctivitis. *Eye (Lond)*. 1990;4(Pt 5):760–764.

[27] Norrman G, Falth-Magnusson K. Adverse reactions to skin prick testing in children – prevalence and possible risk factors. *Pediatr Allergy Immunol*. 2009;20:273–278.

[28] Liccardi G et al. Systemic reactions from skin testing: literature review. *J Investig Allergol Clin Immunol*. 2006;16:75–78.

[29] Steinke JW, Borish RSS. Genetics of allergic disease L. *J. Allergy Clin Immunol*. 2008, 121, 384–87.

[30] Mari A. When does a protein become an allergen? Searching for a dynamic definition based on most advanced technology tools. *Clin Exp Allergy*. 2008, 38, 1089–94.

[31] Bonds RS., Midoro-Horiuti T., Goldblum R. A structural basis for food allergy:the role of cross reactivity. *Curr. Opin. Allergy Clin Immunol*. 2008;8, 82–86.

[32] Sastre J. Molecular diagnosis in allergy. Clin Exp. *Allergy*. 2010: 30, 1–15.

[33] Salcedo G., Diaz-Perales A. Component Resolved Diagnosis of allergy: more is better ? Clin. Exp Allergy 2010; 40, 836-838

[34] Sastre J., Landivar ME: How molecular diagnosis can change allergen-specific immunotherapy prescription in a complex pollen area Allergy 2012 ; 67, 709-711

[35] Canonica GW, Ansotegui IJ, Pawankar R. A WAO - ARIA - GA²LEN consensus document on molecular-based allergy diagnostics. World Allergy Organ J. 2013 Oct 3;6(1):17.

[36] Douladiris N, Savvatianos S, A molecular diagnostic algorithm to guide pollen immunotherapy in southern Europe: towards component-resolved management of allergic diseases. Int Arch Allergy Immunol. 2013;162(2):163-72

[37] Treudler R, Simon JC. Overview of component resolved diagnostics. Curr Allergy Asthma Rep. 2013 Feb;13(1):110-7.

[38] Ciprandi G, Incorvaia C, Puccinelli P. What should drive the choice of allergen for immunotherapy in polysensitized patients? Ann Allergy Asthma Immunol. 2012 Aug;109(2):148-9.

[39] Hatzler L, Panetta V, Lau S et al. Molecular spreading and predictive value of preclinical IgE response to Phleumpratense in children with hay fever. J Allergy Clin Immunol. 2012 Oct;130(4):894-901

[40] Matricardi PM Molecular profile clustering of IgE responses and potential implications for specific immunotherapy. Curr Opin Allergy Clin Immunol. 2013 Aug;13(4): 438-45.

[41] Savi E, Peveri S, Incorvaia C. et al. Association between a low IgE response to Phl p 5 and absence of asthma in patients with grass pollen allergy. Clin Mol Allergy. 2013 Dec 5;11(1):3.

[42] Passalacqua G., Melioli G. The additionalvalues of microarray allergen assay in the management of polysensitized patients with respiratory allergy. Allergy. 2013 Aug; 68(8):1029-33.

[43] Walker SM, Durham SR et al. Immunotherapy for allergic rhinitis. Clin Exp Allergy. 2011 Sep;41(9):1177-200.

[44] Melioli G, Passalacqua G et al. Component-resolved diagnosis in pediatric allergic rhinoconjunctivitis and asthma. Curr Opin Allergy Clin Immunol. 2013 Aug;13(4): 446-51.

[45] Schmid-Grendelmeier P. Recombinant allergens. For routine use or still only science? Hautarzt. 2010 Nov;61(11):946-53.

[46] Ruiz-García M, García Del Potro M et al. Profilin: a relevant aeroallergen? J Allergy Clin Immunol. 2011 Aug;128(2):416-8.

[47] Kespohl S, Maryska S Biochemical and immunological analysis of mould skin prick test solution: current status of standardization. Clin Exp Allergy. 2013 Nov;43(11): 1286-96

[48] Calderón MA1, Casale T et al. Allergen immunotherapy:a new semantic framework from the European Academy of Allergy and Clinical Immunology /American Academy of Allergy Asthma and Immunology/PRACTALL Consensus Report. Allergy. 2013 Jul;68(7):825-8.

[49] Morris DL. WHO position paper on oral (sublingual) immunotherapy. Ann Allergy Asthma Immunol. 1999 Nov;83(5):423-4.

[50] Moingeon P. Update on Immune Mechanisms Associated with Sublingual Immunotherapy:Practical Implications for the Clinician J Allergy Clin Immunol Pract. 2013 May-Jun;1(3):228-41.

[51] Calderon MA, Eichel A, Makatsori M, Pfaar O. Comparability of subcutaneous and sublingual immunotherapy outcomes in allergic rhinitis clinical trials. Curr Opin Allergy Clin Immunol. 2012 Jun;12(3):249-56

[52] Durham SR, Emminger W. SQ-standardized sublingual grass immunotherapy: confirmation of disease modification 2 years after 3 years of treatment in a randomized trial. J Allergy Clin Immunol. 2012 Mar;129(3):717-725

[53] Valovirta E. Design and recruitment for the GAP trial, investigating the preventive effect on asthma development of an SQ-standardized grass allergy immunotherapy tablet in children with grass pollen induced allergic rhinoconjunctivitis. ClinTher. 2011 Oct;33(10):1537-46)

[54] EMA Doc. Ref. CHMP/EWP/18504/2006). London 20 November 200855

[55] Passalacqua G, Melioli G. The additional values of microarray allergen assay in the management ofpolysensitized patients with respiratory allergy. Allergy, 2013, 1-556

[56] Melioli G, Marcomini L et al. The IgE repertoire in children and adolescents resolved at component level: a cross –sectional study. Pediatr. Allergy Immunol 2012: 23, 433-44057

[57] Ciprandi G, Melioli G et al. Immunotherapy in polysensitized patients: new changes for the allergists? Ann Allergy Asthma Immunol 2012:109 392-94

[58] Matricardi P. Molecular profile clustering of IgE responses and potential implications for specific immunotherapy. Curr. Opin. Allergy Clin. Immunol 2013, 13:438-445

[59] Prigione I, Morandi F et al. Interferon –gamma and IL-10 may protect from allergic polysensitization in children: preliminary evidence. Allergy 2010: 65, 740-42

[60] Baiardini I, Bousquet PJ et al. Recommendations for assessing patient-reported outcomes and health-related quality of life in clinical trials on allergy: a GA(2)LEN taskforce position paper. Global Allergy and Asthma European Network. Allergy. 2010 Mar;65(3):290-5

[61] Baiardini I, Braido F et al. Allergic diseases and their impact on quality of life. Ann Allergy Asthma Immunol. 2006 Oct;97(4):419-28

[62] Didier A, Worm M. Sustained 3-year efficacy of pre- and coseasonal 5-grass-pollen sublingual immunotherapy tablets in patients with grass pollen-induced rhinoconjunctivitis. J Allergy Clin Immunol. 2011 Sep;128(3):559-66

[63] Powell RJ, Frew AJ, Corrigan CJ, Durham. SR. Effect of grass pollen immunotherapy with Alutard SQ on quality of life in seasonal allergic rhinoconjunctivitis. Allergy. 2007 Nov;62(11):1335-8

[64] Wessel F, Chartier A. Safety and Tolerability of an SQ_tandardizedGRAss Allergy Immunotherapy Tablet (Grazax) in Real-Life Setting for Three Consecutive Seasons – The GRAAL. Clin Drug Investig. 2012 Jul 1;32(7):451-63

[65] Ariano R, Berto P, Tracci D, Incorvaia C, Frati F. Pharmacoeconomics of allergen immunotherapy compared with symptomatic drug treatment in patients with allergic rhinitis and asthma. Allergy Asthma Proc. 2006 Mar-Apr;27(2):159-63.

[66] Simoens S. The cost-effectiveness of immunotherapy for respiratory allergy: are view. Allergy 2012, 67, 1087-1105

[67] Berto P, Bassi M, Incorvaia C, Frati F Cost cost-effectiveness of sublingual immunotherapy in chidren with allergic rhinitis and asthma Eur. Ann. All. Clin. Immunol 2005- 37, 303-30

[68] Hankin CS, Cox L, Bronstone A, Wang Z. Allergy immunotherapy: Reduced health care costs in adults and children with allergic rhinitis J Allergy Clin Immunol 2013:131 1084-91

[69] Omnes IF, Bousquet J. Pharmacoeconomic assessment of specific immunotherapiy vs current symptomatic treatment for allergic rhinitis and asthma in France. Eur Ann Allergy Clin Immunol. 2007; 39(5):148-56.